Learning About Voice

Vocal Hygiene Activities for Children

A Resource Manual

Learning About Voice
Vocal Hygiene Activities for Children

A Resource Manual

Michael J. Moran, Ph.D.
Professor
Department of Communication Disorders
Auburn University

Elizabeth Zylla-Jones, M.S.
Clinical Instructor
Department of Communication Disorders
Auburn University

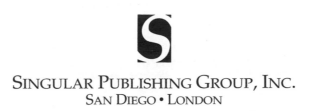

SINGULAR PUBLISHING GROUP, INC.
SAN DIEGO • LONDON

MW

Singular Publishing Group, Inc.
401 West A Street, Suite 325
San Diego, California 92101-7904

Singular Publishing Ltd.
19 Compton Terrace
London N1 2UN, UK

Singular Publishing Group, Inc., publishes textbooks, clinical manuals, clinical reference books, journals, videos, and multimedia materials on speech-language pathology, audiology, otorhinolaryngology, special education, early childhood, aging, occupational therapy, physical therapy, rehabilitation, counseling, mental health, and voice. For your convenience, our entire catalog can be accessed on our website at **http://www.singpub.com.** Our mission to provide you with materials to meet the daily challenges of the ever changing health care/educational environment will remain on course if we are in touch with you. In that spirit, we welcome your feedback on our products. Please telephone **(1-800-521-8545)**, fax **(1-800-774-8398)**, or e-mail **(singpub@mail.cerfnet.com)** your comments and requests to us.

Typeset in 12/14 Palatino by Thompson Type
Printed in the United States of America by McNaughton and Gunn

Library of Congress Cataloging-in-Publication Data
Moran, Michael J., Ph. D.
    Learning about voice : vocal hygiene activities for children /
Michael J. Moran, Elizabeth Zylla-Jones.
        p. cm.
    Includes bibliographical references.
    ISBN 1-56593-942-5 (soft cover : alk. paper)
    1. Voice disorders in children—Rehabilitation. 2. Voice—Care
and hygiene. I. Zylla-Jones, Elizabeth. II. Title.
    [DNLM: 1. Voice—physiology. 2. Voice Disorders—in infancy &
childhood. WV 501 M829L 1998]
RF511.5.M67 1998
618.92'855—dc21
DNLM/DLC
for Library of Congress   98-10016
                                                          CIP

11/21/02 Plus 1 cassette

Contents

Preface

This program was designed with two objectives in mind. The first was to provide a rationale for the use of a vocal hygiene program. Typically, speech-language pathologists are trained to work in one-to-one situations or in small groups until specified criteria are met. An educational, preventative program directed toward a relatively large group over a predetermined time period may not be a comfortable situation for many speech-language pathologists. Therefore, in the first section of this manual, the reader is provided with a discussion of the concept of a vocal hygiene program and with a justification for the use of such an approach.

Our second objective was to provide a variety of suggestions and materials that speech-language pathologists might use to construct and administer vocal hygiene programs. We wanted to describe a program that could easily be adapted for children across a wide range of ages but that would still follow a basic outline and achieve similar objectives regardless of the age of the children to whom it is directed. We also wanted to ensure that the program was flexible enough to allow clinicians to enhance it with their own creativity and to apply it in a variety of settings. In subsequent sections of this manual the stages of our vocal hygiene program are described. In each stage, goals are identified and suggested activities and materials appropriate for various ages and situations are provided. Speech-language pathologists are encouraged to use the suggested activities and materials provided and to supplement the suggested activities with activities of their own creation that are appropriate to the goals of each stage and to the needs of specific children.

Experienced speech-language pathologists will recognize that many of the activities in the various stages of the vocal hygiene program are also appropriate for the early stages of more traditional one-to-one or small group voice therapy. Clinicians are encouraged to modify the goals and activities presented here for use in treatment programs directed toward a variety of voice and resonance problems. The activities suggested in this program would be particularly appropriate for problems stemming from vocal hyperfunction and/or vocal abuse.

We extend sincere thanks to Darlene Houston who helped in many ways in the preparation of this work. We also acknowledge those who provided voice samples and served as models for our photographs: Clay Askew, Jana Borchert, Joseph Burque, Peter Byrne, Morgan Bell, Emlynn Jones, Kevin Moran, Mark Moran, Colin Morrison, Elise Morrison, and Leah Nusbaum. We recognize Delia Duke who created the original poem on which "Willy Owl's Voice Lesson" was based. Finally, we express our appreciation to the very creative person who drew all of the illustrations in this manual but who wishes to remain anonymous. Thanks to all of you.

SECTION

The Concept of a Vocal Hygiene Program

In addition to the evaluation and treatment of communication disorders, speech-language pathologists are concerned with the prevention of such disorders. Among the most preventable communication disorders are the voice problems that result from abuse and misuse of the vocal mechanism. Although this is a preventable problem, the incidence of abuse-related voice disorders among children may be increasing. Senturia and Wilson (1968) reported the prevalence of voice disorders among school-age children to be about 6%. Subsequent studies (Harden, 1986; Mutch, 1976; Sauchelli, 1979) have reported the prevalence of chronic hoarseness in elementary school children to be between 24% and 38%.

How best to deal with problems related to vocal abuse and misuse is not universally agreed on. Moran and Pentz (1987) surveyed 535 otolaryngologists nationwide and reported that more than 59% indicated that voice therapy was the treatment of choice for children with nodules. However, more than 15% responded that "no direct intervention" was the treatment of choice and approximately the same percentage of respondents favored some other form of treatment including counseling the parent and/or the child to reduce vocal abuse.

With regard to elementary school children, Sander (1989) argued that the best treatment for chronic hoarseness might be no treatment at all. The reasons for Sander's suggestion that speech-language pathologists refrain from intervention with chronically hoarse children include the following: Speech-language pathologists often have a very narrow range of acceptability for voice quality differences. As a result children are judged in relation to unreasonably high standards of vocal aesthetics. Sander further stated that many children who experience prolonged hoarseness in the early years develop normal voice quality by puberty. Another point in Sander's argument against intervention for voice disorders in children is that such treatment may make children "phonophobic," that is, fearful of using the voice for any loud talking, coughing, or laughing. Finally, Sander argued that to provide direct treatment to all those elementary school children with chronic hoarseness would result in unmanageable caseloads for the often already overburdened school clinicians.

In direct opposition to Sander (1989), Kahane and Mayo (1989) argued for the aggressive management of voice disorders in children. They based their argument on the following observations: Injury to the voice at an early age may affect the "vitality" of the adult voice. They further pointed to evidence that voice problems observed in many adults reflect a continuation of patterns that originated in childhood. Voice disorders in children may result in social and academic penalties. Kahane and Mayo (1989) cited research involving middle school students that casts doubt on the observation that voice disorders in children are dramatically reduced after elementary school. Finally, Kahane and Mayo (1989) indicated that the majority of otolaryngologists favor some form of voice therapy as the treatment of choice for children with vocal nodules.

Although we agree with Sander (1989) that traditional direct intervention for chronic hoarseness in children would result in unmanageable caseloads, we also agree with Kahane and Mayo (1989) that ignoring the problem is not in the best interest of these children. Speech-language pathologists are faced with a dual challenge in regard to abuse-related voice disorders. First, they should be actively involved in the prevention of this most preventable category of communication disorders. Second, speech-language pathologists may need to develop alternatives to traditional voice therapy to provide services to those who can benefit from such alternative programs while avoiding unmanageable caseloads. Vocal hygiene programs appear to incorporate features that make them a reasonable approach to both the challenge of prevention and that of a more efficient means of treating large numbers of clients.

❖ Vocal hygiene programs are educational and preventative in nature. They are designed to make the recipients more aware of voice and of the potential for the abuse and misuse of voice. The preventative nature of vocal hygiene programs serves a function that traditional voice therapy does not.

❖ In addition to their preventative function, there is some evidence that vocal hygiene programs may improve deviant voice quality (Nilson & Schneiderman, 1983). It is not surprising that vocal hygiene programs could have a therapeutic effect. Vocal hygiene programs target an increased awareness of voice, discrimination of vocal features, and the identification and reduction of vocal abuse. These same objectives are targets in most traditional programs for the treatment of vocal abuse-related disphonias.

❖ Vocal hygiene programs can be administered to large groups. Such group activity has several advantages. Recipients are not singled out as they are in traditional voice therapy programs. The group setting also offers opportunities to learn about other voices, to improve discrimination skills, to share experiences regarding voice usage, and to engage in situational activities that reflect more naturalistic communication (Burk, 1972).

❖ Such programs generally require a finite number of sessions over a brief period of time.

Several vocal hygiene programs have been described in the literature. Some of the more well known include those by Nilson and Schneiderman (1983), Terrell and Morgan (1980), and Cook, Palaski, and Hanson (1979). Each of these programs was designed for a specific age group and offers a fairly limited set of activities. The purpose of this program is to provide speech-language pathologists with an outline for a vocal hygiene program that would be appropriate for children from preschool through junior high school, and to provide numerous suggestions that a clinician may use to plan and implement such a program.

The Purpose of a Vocal Hygiene Program

Regardless of the age group for which a vocal hygiene program is intended, there are certain general goals toward which such programs should be directed. In the program described here, these goals are incorporated into six program stages. These stages are described in the following paragraphs.

STAGE I. Develop an Awareness of Voice

There is an old story about a football coach whose team was not doing well. The coach met with the team and told them that he thought they needed to get back to basics and master the fundamentals of the game. To begin his "back to basics" approach, the coach held up a ball and said, "Men, this is a football." Using that old coach's approach to teaching basics, we need to begin our vocal hygiene programs by demonstrating what voice is. This can be accomplished in many ways. In the program described here, we incorporate two goals into this first stage. The first goal is to enable group members to identify others based solely on speech samples. We provide several suggested activities for accomplishing this goal. These suggested activities involve people in the group, familiar school personnel, celebrities, tape recordings, telephone, TV, radio, CDs, and tapes.

After accomplishing the first goal, it is frequently necessary to focus attention on the voice as separate from the other features of an individual's speech pattern. Many children have difficulty at first separating voice from other aspects of speech such as articulation, rate, and fluency. Therefore our second goal is to distinguish voice from other speech characteristics. The suggested activities provided for this goal later in this manual will help the members of any vocal hygiene group make such a distinction.

STAGE II. Develop a Rudimentary Understanding of Where and How the Voice is Produced

Some basic knowledge of the vocal mechanism and how that mechanism functions to produce voice can be quite helpful in understanding common voice disorders and the vocal abuse that causes those disorders. Although the vocabulary and degree of detail will vary greatly with different groups, it is not necessary to provide more than a brief description of the vocal mechanism for any vocal hygiene group. Keep in mind, however, that no matter how brief or basic the information may be, it must be accurate. The basic elements of a description of the vocal mechanism include:

1. Identifying the larynx as the source of phonation.
2. Locating the larynx.
3. Describing the structure and function of the larynx in producing voice.

These basic elements constitute the goals for Stage II in our program. In the following section, we provide suggestions for various levels of explanation regarding the vocal mechanism and a number of diagrams and drawings at various levels of sophistication.

STAGE III. Identify and Label Various Vocal Parameters

Once the individual's attention has been focused on voice, the instructor must be able to call attention to various vocal parameters. By isolating aspects such as pitch, loudness, and various voice qualities, the group may be led to focus on specific parameters of the voice rather than viewing voice as a poorly understood entity. Once the members of the group are familiar with these vocal parameters, learning to vary them further reinforces the students' awareness.

STAGE IV. Develop Discrimination Skill

Eventually, the students must be able to monitor their own voice. They must develop some facility to distinguish variations within the selected vocal parameters. How severe is the hoarseness in a particular sample? Is the pitch of one voice sample higher or lower than another sample? Is one voice inappropriately loud while another is too soft? It is not necessary, or even desirable, that all vocal hygiene students use professional terms to identify and describe these features. As Burk (1972) suggested, each group may select a different set of terms with which to describe voice features, but the different terms represent "their language" for talking about voice features and therefore are more meaningful. What is necessary is that the group members use the terms they decide on consistently and that the clinician and all group members share the same understanding of the terms.

STAGE V. Identify and Reduce Vocal Abuse and Misuse

Perhaps the most important portion of a vocal hygiene program is the identification and reduction of vocal abuse. Too often vocal abuse is inadequately described simply as "yelling and screaming." There are at least two problems with such an oversimplified explanation. First, the difference between yelling and screaming has never been entirely clear to us. More important, this description presents a fairly narrow view of the various vocal behaviors that can be abusive. We propose that the following goals should be accomplished in order to identify and reduce vocal abuse. First, familiarize students with the nature of vocal abuse. What is vocal abuse? Which activities or behaviors are considered vocally abusive? Next, teach the students to identify vocal abuse in others. Once they are able to identify vocal abuse in other speakers, the students should identify their own patterns of vocal abuse. Once these goals are achieved, alternatives to vocally abusive behaviors can be suggested. Finally, any vocal abuse exhibited by members of the group should be reduced in a systematic manner. This last goal needs to be an ongoing process after the formal portion of the vocal hygiene program has ended. Remember, a vocal hygiene program is essentially an educational and preventative program provided over a short and finite period of time. It would not be practical to spend the same amount of time on the elimination of abuses that a clinician may spend in a traditional program of voice therapy.

Keeping the above caveat in mind, we do believe that the identification and reduction of vocal abuse is the essence of any vocal hygiene program. Therefore we have provided many suggested activities to achieve the goals of this stage. Keep in mind that the activities in this program are suggestions. Clinicians should choose those which they feel most appropriate for their particular groups. It is not expected that the clinician use every activity.

STAGE VI. Summarize and Facilitate Carryover

In order to ensure that the group members have understood and retained critical information from the previous stages of the program, it is desirable to reserve some time to review the most important aspects of the program before disbanding the group. It is also often desirable to provide some token reward to the group members for completing the program and to provide some tangible reminders concerning appropriate and inappropriate voice usage. The review of important points can take the form of a summary, quiz, group discussion, or other activity. Rewards may be certificates of completion, ribbons, or buttons. Reminders may include providing the group members with handouts, notebooks, or small posters listing vocal do's and don'ts or contracts to use the voice in an appropriate fashion.

Outline of the Vocal Hygiene Program

Stages and Goals

For each of the six program stages described previously we have identified several goals. The stages and goals are presented here in outline form:

    I. **Develop an Awareness of Voice**

        A. **Identify others based on speech samples**

        B. **Distinguish voice from other speech characteristics**

    II. **Develop a Rudimentary Understanding of the Vocal Mechanism**

        A. **Identify, locate, and feel the larynx vibrate**

        B. **Describe the structure and function of the larynx**

   III. **Identify and Label Various Voice Parameters**

      A. **Pitch**

      B. **Loudness**

      C. **Quality**

   IV. **Develop Discrimination Skills**

      A. **Discriminate appropriate/inappropriate pitch**

      B. **Discriminate appropriate/inappropriate loudness**

      C. **Discriminate adequate/inadequate quality**

      D. **Identify inappropriate/inadequate vocal parameters**

   V. **Identify and Reduce Vocal Abuse**

      A. **Familiarize students with the nature of vocal abuse**

      B. **Identify vocal abuse in others**

      C. **Identify the vocal abuse patterns of each group member**

      D. **Suggest alternatives to vocal abuse**

      E. **Reduce vocal abuse in a systematic manner**

   VI. **Summarize and Facilitate Carryover**

      A. **Review important points**

      B. **Provide reminders for the appropriate use of voice**

      C. **Provide rewards for completion of the program**

We believe that these program stages and the accompanying goals are appropriate in most all situations and broad enough to apply to a wide range of ages. Therefore we suggest that these should form the basic structure of a vocal hygiene program. **The stages and goals, which are identified by boldface type in the outlines in this section and throughout the text, should be applied to all groups regardless of age or level of understanding about voice.**

To achieve the goals in these six stages, clinicians may use any number of procedures and activities. Those procedures and activities will be different for different groups and depend on such factors as age, level of awareness of voice, setting, and time constraints, just to name a few. In the outline that follows and throughout the remainder of this manual, we identify broadly defined *procedures* that may be used by the clinician to achieve each of the goals, and we suggest numerous specific *activities* for each procedure. The procedures and activities appear in bold italic type in the following outline and in the text that follows in order to contrast them with the bold-faced stages and goals. Unlike the stages and goals, which clinicians should incorporate into each vocal hygiene program, the suggested procedures and activities are just that, suggestions. Clinicians may choose those procedures and activities that they feel to be appropriate for a particular vocal hygiene group. Clinicians may, and in fact are encouraged to, add their own procedures and activities as they see fit under each of the boldfaced goals. In this way, the program provides both structure and flexibility.

The complete vocal hygiene program that we have designed, including stages, goals, procedures, and activities, is outlined below. Remember the outline, and the discussion to follow, is organized as follows:

I. One of the Six Stages of the Program

    A. A specific goal for achieving the major purpose

        1. A broadly stated procedure for meeting the goal

            a. A suggested specific activity for the procedure

The remainder of the text will be a detailed discussion of the goals, procedures, and activities for each stage.

Outline of the program including stages, goals, procedures and activities.

I. Develop an Awareness of Voice

    A. Identify others based on speech samples

        1. People in the group

            a. live voice samples

            b. tape recorded samples

        2. School personnel

            a. tape recorded samples

            b. live voice activity (Mystery Guest)

            c. imitations

        3. Celebrities

            a. identify from taped samples

            b. match pictures to taped samples

            c. think of celebrities with distinctive voices

        4. Family members

            a. tape activity (Guess the family member)

            b. tape activity (Who's family?)

            c. telephone activity

    B. Distinguish voice from other speech characteristics

        1. Distinguish voice from speech

            a. whisper

            b. humming

            c. talking with mouth closed

         2. Distinguish voice from articulation problems

            a. tape recorded demonstration

            b. clinician simulation

      c. backward play tape activity

      d. contrast activity

   3. Distinguish voice from fluency

      a. clinician simulation

      b. tape recorded demonstration

      c. contrast activity

   4. Distinguish voice from accent patterns

      a. tape recorded demonstration

      b. live voice activity

II. Develop a Rudimentary Understanding of the Vocal Mechanism

  A. Identify the larynx as the site of production and locate the structure.

    1. Simple explanation

      a. Adam's apple

      b. diagrams and drawings

    2. Physically locate the larynx and feel it vibrate

      a. place finger on larynx

      b. feel vibration during phonation

    3. Contrasting the feel of the larynx during voiced and voiceless productions

      a. voiced and voiceless continuants

      b. kazoo

      c. instrumentation

  B. Describe the structure and function of the larynx and vocal folds

    1. Diagrams, drawings, videos, models

      a. drawings with program

      b. drawings from other sources

      c. videos

      d. models

    2. Analogies

      a. rubber bands

      b. musical instruments

    3. Games

      a. coloring pages

      b. word search

      c. crossword puzzles

      d. scrambled word puzzles

III. **Identify and Label Various Vocal Parameters**

  A. **Identify and vary pitch**

    1. Introduce concept of pitch with nonvocal sounds

      a. pure-tone audiometer

      b. musical instruments

      c. using word pairs

      d. students generate list of objects associated with high and low pitched sound

      e. word search

      f. crossword puzzle

      g. scrambled word puzzle

    2. Demonstrate vocal pitch variations

      a. tape recorded samples

      b. clinician demonstration

      c. group members as examples

    3. Students vary their pitch

      a. sing the scale

      b. climb and descend the pitch ladder

      c. talk in the lowest/highest possible pitch

      d. talk like a man/woman

      e. use instrumentation for feedback

  B. **Identify and provide examples of loudness**

    1. Introduce the concept of loudness with nonvocal sounds

      a. pure-tone audiometer

      b. radio

      c. word pairs

      d. students generate suggestions of loud and soft sounds

      e. word search

      f. crossword puzzle

      g. scrambled word puzzle

    2. Demonstrate vocal loudness variations

      a. tape recorded examples

      b. clinician demonstration

      c. group members as examples

      d. group member drawings

      e. describe people who use loud/quiet voices

3. Students vary their loudness

    a. talk softly (not whispering) then talk louder (not yelling)

    b. climb and descend the loudness ladder

    c. use instrumentation for feedback; discuss when we use loud/quiet voice

    d. discuss situational loudness

    e. role play situational loudness

C. Identify and provide examples of various voice qualities

1. Demonstrate variations of vocal hyperfunction (tense), hypofunction (breathy), hoarseness, and hard glottal attacks

    a. clinician simulation

    b. tape recorded examples

2. Use group members

    a. simulation

    b. group members as examples

IV. Develop Discrimination Skills

A. Distinguish appropriate/inappropriate pitch

1. Live voice activities

    a. clinician simulation

    b. group simulation

2. Matching voice samples to pictures

    a. female or child

    b. adult male

    c. animal or object

    d. various ages and genders

    e. various animals or objects

3. Tape recorded speech samples

    a. presentation of various pitch levels

B. Distinguish appropriate/inappropriate loudness

1. Live voice activities

    a. clinician simulation

    b. group simulation

2. Matching voice samples to pictures

    a. quiet setting

    b. normal conversation

    c. various activities

    3. Discuss situational loudness

      a. group discussion

      b. quiz

    4. Tape recorded speech samples

      a. presentation of various loudness levels

C. Identify inadequate voice quality (breathy, harsh, hoarse)

    1. Live voice

      a. clinician simulation

      b. use group members

    2. Taped voice samples

      a. identify specific voice qualities

      b. identify various voice qualities

D. Identify inappropriate vocal parameters

    1. Live voice activities

      a. clinician simulation

    2. Tape recorded activities

      a. use a voice profile

      b. celebrity voices

      c. disordered voices

      d. name that voice

V. Identify and Reduce Vocal Abuse

  A. Familiarize students with the nature of vocal abuse

    1. Define and provide specific examples

      a. simple description

      b. vocal abuse checklist

      c. poster of "America's most unwanted vocal behaviors"

      d. pictures of children engaged in vocal abuse

      e. poem

      f. puppet show

      g. crossword

      h. word search

      i. scrambled word puzzle

      j. hangman

      k. vocal abuse pictionary

    2. Identify situations that contribute to vocal abuse

      a. list situations

  b. group generates list

  c. group selects situations

 B. Identify vocal abuse in others

  1. Identify abusive behaviors from photos and drawings

   a. pictures of quiet and loud activities

   b. drawing abusive and nonabusive behaviors

   c. categorizing behaviors

  2. Identify abuse from audio and videotapes

   a. rock singers

   b. television characters

   c. children at play

   d. role playing

 C. Identify vocal abuse patterns of group members

  1. Self-evaluation

   a. vocal abuse inventory

   b. self-monitoring

  2. Involve others

   a. abuse monitors

   b. voice buddies

   c. tape record group members

 D. Suggest alternatives to vocally abusive behavior

  1. Clinician suggestions

   a. list

  2. Group generated alternatives

   a. each member makes suggestions

   b. group suggestions for selected members

   c. stories

   d. puppet show/skit

 E. Chart and reduce abuse

  1. Establish a baseline

   a. use a small note pad

   b. audio or videotape group members

  2. Target specific behaviors to be reduced

   a. group members select target behavior

   b. clinician selects target behavior

      3. Involve others in abuse reduction

         a. ask parents and/or teachers

         b. request for assistance form

         c. chart abuses

         d. use "good voice reminders"

         e. use a token economy

         f. use a contract

VI. Summarize and Facilitate Carryover

    A. Reiterate important points

      1. Clinician reviews major points

         a. oral summary

         b. follow the outline

      2. Review by quizzing the group

         a. use the list of questions provided

         b. clinician constructs quiz

    B. Provide tangible reminders for the appropriate use of voice

      1. Use a notebook

         a. 10-easy steps

         b. list of do's and don'ts

         c. do and don't pictures

         d. each member makes a personal list

         e. 10-step outline

      2. Develop a contract

         a. use a list of abusive behaviors

         b. extend previous contracts

    C. Provide rewards for completion of the program

      1. Provide mementos of completion

         a. certificates

         b. buttons

         c. ribbons

      2. Use activities to mark completion

         a. a good voice party

         b. a trip to the theater

SECTION

Procedures and Activities for a Vocal Hygiene Program

In this section the procedures and activities listed for each of the goals in the preceding outline will be described in detail. Once again, we suggest that clinicians target all of the essential elements of the program regardless of the age of the group or the setting. **These essential elements are the stages and goals in boldface type in the preceding outline and in the following section.** The broadly defined procedures and specific activities, in standard type, are suggestions that clinicians may choose to use based on the specific target group and/or setting. Clinicians are encouraged to use additional activities that they feel would be appropriate for their specific groups. These additional activities, however, should fit the essential elements of the program. The remainder of this section is organized according to the outline presented earlier. This organization allows the reader to move easily from the outline to the detailed description of activities and from any activity back to the outline. For example, for an activity identified as *Activity II.B.1.a.* the Roman numeral refers to the major stage. The upper-case letter refers to the goal. The Arabic numeral refers to the procedure and the lower-case letter identifies the specific activity.

Tape Recordings and Photographs

Many of the activities described in the following section involve tape recorded speech samples and photographs. We have provided a tape recording to accompany this manual. The activities for which the taped samples may be used are indicated in the text by a **T**. We have also included 21 photographs that can be used for various activities. These photographs may be found at the end of the manual. Activities for which the photographs may be used are indicated in the text by a **P.** In some cases the clinician may choose from several photographs that fit a specific activity. The taped samples and photographs provided are suggested materials. The clinician should feel free to use any or all of these materials or to supply other tape samples and photos.

STAGE

Develop an Awareness of Voice

Individuals with voice disorders often are aware of their voice by the time they see a speech-language pathologist. They are concerned about the way their voice sounds or report that other people have commented on their voice. Students in a vocal hygiene program, on the other hand, typically have never given much thought to voice—theirs or that of anyone else. Many people tend to confuse voice with other aspects of speech such as accent, rate, or even articulation.

The first step in a vocal hygiene program then should focus the attention of the students on the voice. At this early stage of the program the focus need not, and probably should not, be on the individual's own voice, but on the voices of people he or she knows or hears frequently. With young children, this stage may be begun by focusing on the sounds made by animals. The purpose is to demonstrate that everyone has a voice that makes him or her sound different. The voice can be a clue to the gender, age, and emotional state of the person. Many resources can be employed to create activities that will help to develop an awareness of voice. Some suggestions are offered here; most of the activities described can be adjusted according to the age level of the group.

The overall objective of this first stage of the program is to make the students more aware of voice. The following goals should be targeted.

GOAL I.A. Students will identify other speakers based on speech samples only

At this point, the task is to reinforce the idea that everyone sounds different. We are not yet concerned about the distinction between speech and voice. However, speech samples chosen for the activities to achieve this goal should not contain distinctive speech characteristics such as obvious articulation problems, accents, or fluency disorders.

Procedure I.A.1. Using people in the group

This first stage of the program lends itself particularly well to groups as everyone in the group brings a unique voice which can be sampled and discussed.

Activity I.A.1.a. Select two people from the group. Have them introduce themselves and say something about themselves. Next, have the group members close their eyes. Tap one of the selected speakers and have him/her say/read a short utterance. Ask the group who is speaking. The group should be able to identify the speaker with ease. Ask the group how they knew who was speaking. Direct the responses of the group toward the fact that one speaker sounds different from the other. Repeat with other group members as speakers.

Activity I.A.1.b. Tape record the voices of each member of the group. Randomly play back the speech samples and have the group guess who is speaking.

Procedure I.A.2. Using school personnel

In a school setting, students encounter many people, each of whom has a unique voice. These people, who include teachers, administrators, nurses, coaches, custodians, bus drivers, and others, may be used as examples of the variety of human voices.

Activity I.A.2.a. Tape record the principal, teachers of the students in the group, and/or other well known members of the school community. Ask the children to identify the speakers from tape.

Activity I.A.2.b. Have school personnel appear as "Mystery Guests" in the classroom. The "guests" may stand behind a door or a partition or the students may be asked to close their eyes. The "guests" should produce utterances of increasing length until someone in the group can identify the speaker.

Activity I.A.2.c. Ask the group to imitate the voice of one of the school's staff. Have the other members try to guess who each student is imitating. The clinician should guide the group in this activity to attempt to focus on the voice characteristics of the person being imitated rather than on other speech or physical characteristics.

Procedure I.A.3. Using celebrities

Many of our better known entertainers, politicians, news anchors, and other celebrities have very distinctive voices. Cartoon characters and muppets also include very distinctive voices as part of their character. These celebrities can be used to help the group focus on voice.

Activity I.A.3.a. Supply or have the students bring tape recordings, videotapes, or CDs of celebrities with distinctive voices. No tapes of celebrities are provided with this program for two reasons: First, celebrity is a fleeting quality, any of today's familiar voices may be unknown in a few years. (We have received many blank stares from current undergraduate students when we tried to use as a reference the voices of Nelson Rockefeller, Janis Joplin, or Wally Cox.) A second reason is the rather complex copyright laws governing the use of recorded entertainment material. Have the group listen to the recordings and try to identify the speaker. The clinician may wish to focus on some outstanding features of the voices of these celebrities. For example, after listening to James Earl Jones, the clinician may say, "He is easy to recognize because his voice is so deep and powerful."

Activity I.A.3.b. Cut out pictures of famous people from newspapers and magazines and obtain tape samples of these people from newscasts and other media avenues. Have students match tape recorded samples to the pictures.

Activity I.A.3.c. Ask the group to name five famous people (or characters) who have distinctive voices. What is it about the voice of each of these people that makes their voice unique?

Procedure I.A.4. Using family members

Just as each child in the group has a distinctive voice, they each have family members who also can provide examples of the wide range of normal voice.

Activity I.A.4.a. Have children tape record a speech sample from their mother, father, sister, brother, cousin, and so forth. Have the children introduce the relatives (via the tape recorded sample) to the rest of the group. Play a game to see which members of the group can identify the family members of the other children. Ask questions such as, "How did you know that that was Billy's father and not his sister?"

Activity I.A.4.b. Randomly play the tape recordings of family members provided by the children. Select children in the group and ask, "Is this a member of your family?" Then ask how they knew it was or was not a member of their family.

Activity I.A.4.c. Have each child in the group call his/her home and identify the person who answers the phone. Ask how the student knew who it was answering the phone.

GOAL I.B. Students will distinguish speech characteristics from voice characteristics

For this goal, the speech-language pathologist must guide the students in distinguishing between speech and voice. Even adults without specialized training frequently confuse speech features such as articulation errors, accent, or dialectal differences with voice features. It would be beneficial for the work that lies ahead to help the students to focus on voice early in the program.

Procedure I.B.1. Distinguish voice from speech

Show how the group members can make speech without voice and voice without speech.

Activity I.B.1.a. Have the students whisper. Be sure that they are actually whispering and not just speaking with very quiet phonation. Point out that the students are saying words, they are speaking. There is no voice present, however.

Activity I.B.1.b. Have the students hum *Happy Birthday* or some other familiar song. Point out that they are using their voice but there are no words, no speech is being produced.

Activity I.B.1.c. Instruct some of the students to try to talk without opening their mouth. Have others try to understand what the "closed mouth" speakers are saying. Then have the students switch roles. Emphasize how hard it was to produce speech without opening the mouth. Then ask students to produce voice without opening their mouth (hum). Emphasize how easy it was to produce voice in this condition.

Procedure I.B.2. Distinguish voice from articulation disorders

T   *Activity I.B.2.a.* Play tapes of children and adults with articulation disorders but normal voice. Point out to the students the sounds that are in error and ask them to listen to the speech problem then ask them to listen again to the tape but listen only to the voice. (Note: It is important here that the taped examples demonstrate normal voice quality. Many children with articulation errors might also have accompanying voice problems. Such speakers would not be helpful for this activity.)

T   *Activity I.B.2.b.* The clinician can present tape recorded or live simulations of articulation problems, pointing out how his or her voice is the same when he or she makes certain sounds incorrectly. For young children the articulation errors should be limited to one sound and be quite obvious.

T   *Activity I.B.2.c.* Using a tape recorded or live presentation, the clinician should provide speech samples that differ only in articulation proficiency and samples that differ only in some aspect of voice. After presenting each pair of speech samples the clinician should ask, "Are these different in voice or in speech?" For example: Keeping your voice quality, pitch, and loudness as similar as possible, produce the following two sentences.

"We found a kitty cat under our Christmas tree."

versus

"We found a titty tat under our titmas tee."

Then ask, "Were those sentences different in voice or in speech?" Next, repeat the following sentence twice, once in your normal pitch and once in a higher or lower pitch.

"Learning about voice is fun."

Then ask, "Were those sentences different in voice or speech?"

Activity I.B.2.d. Select group members to produce sentences differing in articulation or voice. Ask the rest of the group to listen and determine whether the difference between the two utterances was a speech difference or a voice difference. Some children may become confused and unintentionally change both articulation and voice. This can serve as a challenge for the rest of the group to determine how many realize that the change was made in both areas.

Procedure I.B.3. Distinguish voice from fluency disorders

For most groups this procedure needs only to be targeted briefly. The instructor should simply mention that some people may get stuck on some words when they talk and this is not a voice problem (theories about the continuity between stuttering and spasmodic dysphonia aside). The instructor should then use one or more of the following activities to provide a concrete example.

T **Activity I.B.3.a.** The clinician should make a tape recording or a live presentation in which part or whole word repetitions and/or prolongations are exhibited. The clinician should point out to the group that these disfluencies are speech features and not voice features.

T **Activity I.B.3.b.** Tape recordings of children or adults who stutter may be played for the class to demonstrate fluency problems and to help distinguish them from voice disorders.

T **Activity I.B.3.c.** Using tape recordings or live simulation, the clinician should produce speech samples that differ only in some aspect of voice and samples that differ only in fluency. He or she should then ask the children, "Are these different in voice or in speech?" For example: Keeping your voice quality, pitch, and loudness as similar as possible, produce these two sentences:

"We are reading a funny story."

versus

"We we we are re re re reading a fffffunny story."

Then ask, "Were these sentences different in voice or speech?" Next, repeat the following sentence twice, once at your normal loudness level then again at a much higher or lower loudness.

"I like to eat ice cream."

Then ask, "Were those sentences different in voice or speech?"

Procedure I.B.4. Distinguish voice from accent patterns/dialectal differences

This procedure may be of more or less importance depending on the geographic location of the group. In some geographic regions children are exposed to many different accents or dialectal patterns, such as in large and diverse cities like Los Angeles or New York. In other parts of the country there may be two primary accent or dialectal patterns such as in south central Pennsylvania where Standard English and the Germanic dialect known as Pennsylvania Dutch coexist. In still other areas, Standard English may be the only dialectal pattern used within hundreds of miles. If children do not hear dialectal patterns different from their own there may not be a need to spend much time on this procedure.

Activity I.B.4.a. The clinician may play tapes of speakers with accents or dialectal patterns, pointing out that these are not voice problems. Good sources for such tapes are news programs (especially local news where area residents may be interviewed), local call-in shows, and sports interviews. Video movie rentals and comedy albums on CD or cassette tapes often provide examples of various accents or dialectal patterns.

Activity I.B.4.b. In areas where regional dialects are prevalent, there are likely to be many professionals in the school system or in the community who have become very adept at "style shifting" or "code switching," that is, changing from one dialect to another depending on the situation. Many speech-language pathologists may have skill in this area. These speakers may be asked to provide tape recorded speech samples produced in one dialectal pattern then in another. The children in the group could then be asked if these samples differed in voice or speech as in activities I.B.2.d. and I.B.3.c.

STAGE

Develop a Rudimentary Understanding of the Vocal Mechanism

Regardless of the age group to which a vocal hygiene program is directed, a basic understanding of how voice is produced should prove useful. Such an understanding makes it easier for the students to learn how the voice can be abused and why some of the techniques we will teach are helpful. There is no need to teach a college level anatomy class. However, no matter how simplified it may be, the information presented must be accurate and must contribute to an understanding of the vocal mechanism. The goals of this stage of the program should include teaching the location of the larynx and some minimal information about how that structure functions to produce voice.

Note: Prior to beginning work on this stage, the clinician should consider the level of vocabulary to be used. Many older children will be able to use terms such as "larynx," "vocal folds," and "trachea" with no problem. For younger children terms such as "voicebox," "vocal cords," and "windpipe" may enhance learning. Whenever possible, decisions on vocabulary level should be made by the clinician in consultation with teachers of the group members as the school curriculum may have already included some of this terminology.

GOAL II.A. Identify the larynx as the site of voice production and locate that structure

Procedure II.A.1. Provide a simple explanation of the location of the larynx

Activity II.A.1.a. Use familiar anatomical landmarks to describe the location of the larynx. Most students will know where the Adam's apple is and that can provide a location.

Activity II.A.1.b. Use diagrams to show where in the neck the larynx is located. Diagrams with different levels of detail are shown in Figures 2–1 through 2–5.

Procedure II.A.2. Have the students physically locate the larynx and feel it vibrate during phonation

Activity II.A.2.a. Have each student gently place a finger on his or her Adam's apple. Some students may need the clinician to help with the placement of a finger on the larynx.

Activity II.A.2.b. With the students each holding a finger on the laryngeal area have them hum and feel the vibration.

Procedure II.A.3. Contrast the way the larynx feels during the production of voiced and unvoiced sounds

Activity II.A.3.a. With a finger on the larynx, have students feel the difference between a prolonged voiced sound such as /z/ and a prolonged voiceless sound such as /s/.

Activity II.A.3.b. Have each student construct a makeshift kazoo using a piece of waxed paper folded over a comb. Have them hum a tune so they may feel that the vibration associated with voicing carries through the vocal tract. Then have them blow gently onto the kazoo and note that there is now no sound produced.

Activity II.A.3.c. Many speech-language pathologists may have access to instrumentation such as the Kay Elemetrics Visi-Pitch or the IBM Speech Viewer. These instruments provide visual feedback that will help a child distinguish between voiced and unvoiced sounds.

GOAL II.B. Describe the larynx and how the vocal folds vibrate to produce voice

Procedure II.B.1. Use drawings, diagrams, photos, and videos to illustrate the structures of the larynx and their function in voice

Activity II.B.1.a. Using drawings supplied with the program, the clinician can point out the various structures of the larynx and explain how the air from the lungs vibrates the vocal folds. Some of the accompanying illustrations are more detailed and complex than others. The clinician should select illustrations according to the age of the group. (See Figures 2–1 to 2–5 and Figures 2–6 through 2–9).

Activity II.B.1.b. Illustrations of the laryngeal structure are available from a number of sources in addition to this program. Most speech-language pathologists have several texts that display laryngeal structures. These may be used with older groups.

Activity II.B.1.c. For older children, videotape presentations of the vocal folds during phonation may be quite helpful and interesting. There are several such videotapes commercially available. One tape that provides excellent views is that provided by

Stasney (1996). Also, many otolaryngologists routinely make videotapes of fiberoptic endoscopic and stroboscopic examinations of their patients. The clinician may be able to solicit such videos from cooperative local otolaryngologists.

Activity II.B.1.d. Some clinicians may have models of the larynx available to them. These three dimensional models, which can be handled by the group and viewed from different perspectives, can be quite helpful in explaining the laryngeal structures.

Procedure II.B.2. Use analogies to explain the action of the vocal folds

Activity II.B.2.a. Use a thick rubber band as a rough analogy of the vocal folds. Place each end of the rubber band between the thumb and index finger of each hand. Then blow through the two layers of the rubber band to demonstrate how air sets the band into motion. Stretch the rubber band to show how increasing the length and tension affects pitch.

Activity II.B.2.b. Use a stringed instrument such as a guitar, banjo, or a piano to demonstrate how vibration of the string creates sound; thicker strings create lower pitch, and altering the length of the vibrating portion of the string affects the pitch. One must be careful not to carry the analogy of a vibrating string and vocal fold vibration too far. We do not wish to give the impression that the vocal folds resemble the strings of a guitar. The analogy does work to help convey the idea that length and mass changes affect pitch.

Procedure II.B.3. Use games to reinforce the learning of the previous material

Activity II.B.3.a. Have students color pictures of the larynx which accompany the program. Each of the major structures you wish to emphasize should be colored a different shade. Figures 2–6 and 2–7 may be used for this activity.

Activity II.B.3.b. Have students find the terms listed in the word search found at the end of this section in order to familiarize them with the terminology.

Activity II.B.3.c. Have students solve the crossword puzzle found at the end of this section in order to help associate the names with structures.

Activity II.B.3.d. Have the students complete the scrambled word puzzle at the end of this stage to help familiarize them with terminology.

Word Search Activity for Activity II.B.3.b.

Find the following words (they may be across, down, or diagonal, backward or forward).

Adam's apple
Cartilage
Hum
Larynx

Muscles
Neck
Vibrate
Vocal fold

Voice
Voice box
Whisper

```
L A R M V O M S U E V
V D S E L C S U M Y O
O A V I B R A T E M C
I M X N Y R A L S D L
C S L R A X O Y L V X
E A C N A P P O V N G
B P W A V O F X H E Y
O P H V R L E C I C A
X L W H A T E R S K C
L E M C P M I Y X O L
A D O N P X U L S I H
C V M V O I C E A L R
O E U C X V R A C G Y
I X H R E P S I H W E
```

Answers for Word Search Activity for Activity II.B.3.b.

Find the following words (they may be across, down, or diagonal, backward or forward).

Adam's apple   Muscles   Voice
Cartilage   Neck   Voice box
Hum   Vibrate   Whisper
Larynx   Vocal fold

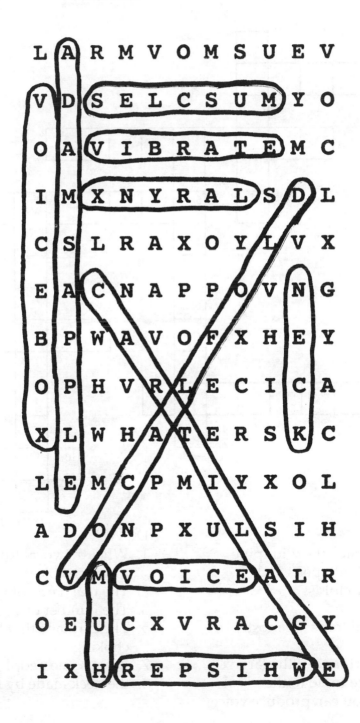

CROSSWORD PUZZLE

Anatomy

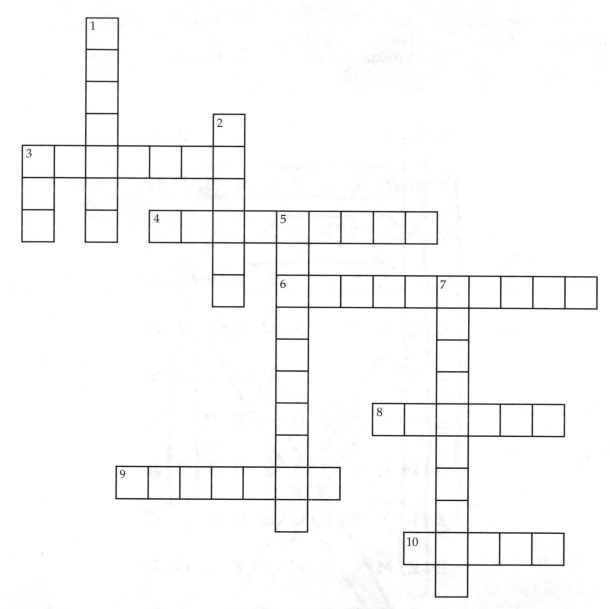

ACROSS:
3. Another name for the windpipe
4. The cartilage that opens and closes the vocal folds
6. Breathing in
8. What the vocal folds are mostly made of
9. The largest cartilage of the larynx
10. What you have to do to the vocal folds before you can produce voice

DOWN:
1. What the vocal folds do when you produce voice
2. The real name of the voice box
3. The number of vocal folds we have
5. The cartilage that helps prevent choking
7. What some people call the bulge in the neck made by the larynx

CROSSWORD PUZZLE

Anatomy

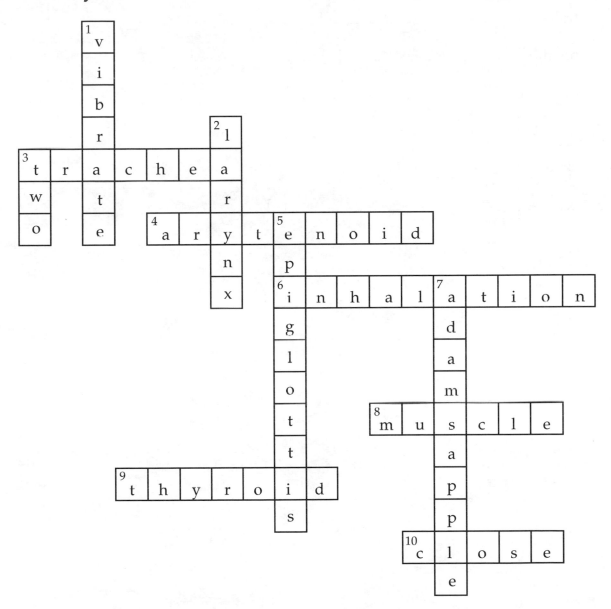

ACROSS:
3. Another name for the windpipe
4. The cartilage that opens and closes the vocal folds
6. Breathing in
8. What the vocal folds are mostly made of
9. The largest cartilage of the larynx
10. What you have to do to the vocal folds before you can produce voice

DOWN:
1. What the vocal folds do when you produce voice
2. The real name of the voice box
3. The number of vocal folds we have
5. The cartilage that helps prevent choking
7. What some people call the bulge in the neck made by the larynx

Scrambled Word Puzzle for Activity II.B.3.d.

Unscramble the following words to find the hidden message. Use the bracketed letters to decode the message.

1. tralceagi   _ _ _ _ _ [_] _ _ _

2. revaitb   _ _ _ _ [_] _ _

3. hripews   _ _ _ _ _ _ [_]

4. nogsrtogloitaloy   _ _ _ _ _ _ [_] _ _ _ _ _ _ _ _ _

5. ckne   [_] _ _ _

6. ixvobeco   _ _ _ _ _ _ _ [_]

Message: _ _ _ _ _ _

KEY: Word Scramble

1. carti[l]age

2. vibr[a]te

3. whispe[r]

4. otolar[y]ngologist

5. [n]eck

6. voicebo[x]

Message: <u>l</u> <u>a</u> <u>r</u> <u>y</u> <u>n</u> <u>x</u>

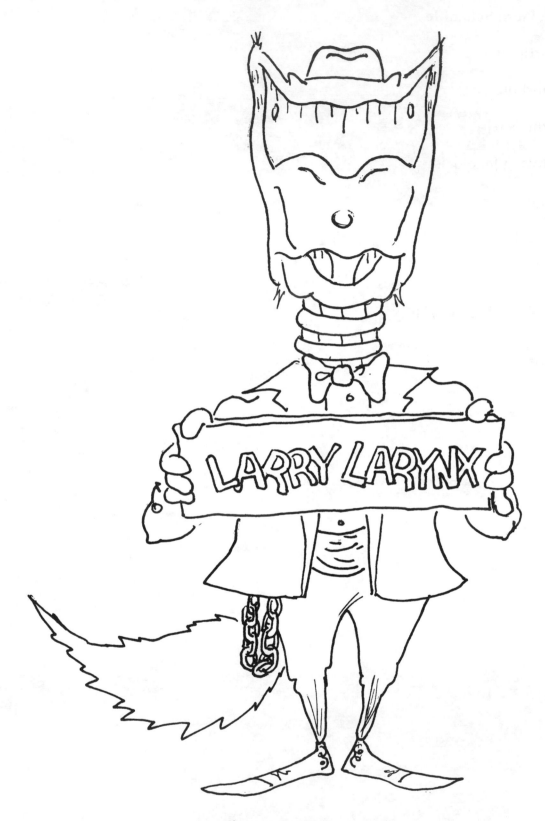

Figure 2–1.

Larry Larynx. An animated figure with a larynx head.

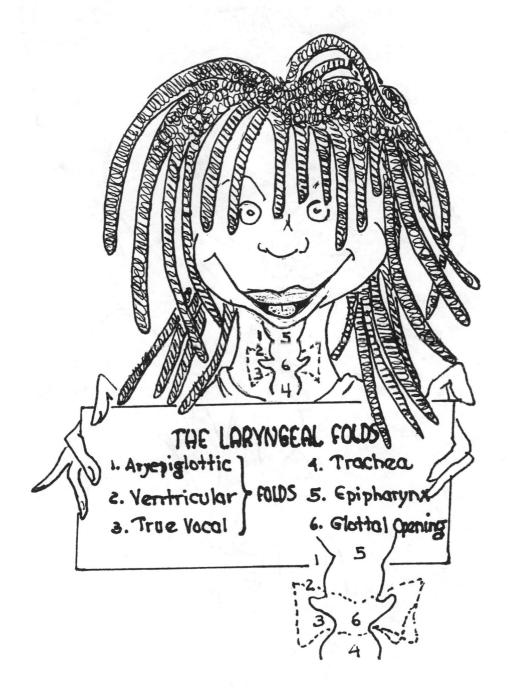

Figure 2–2.
Location of the larynx.

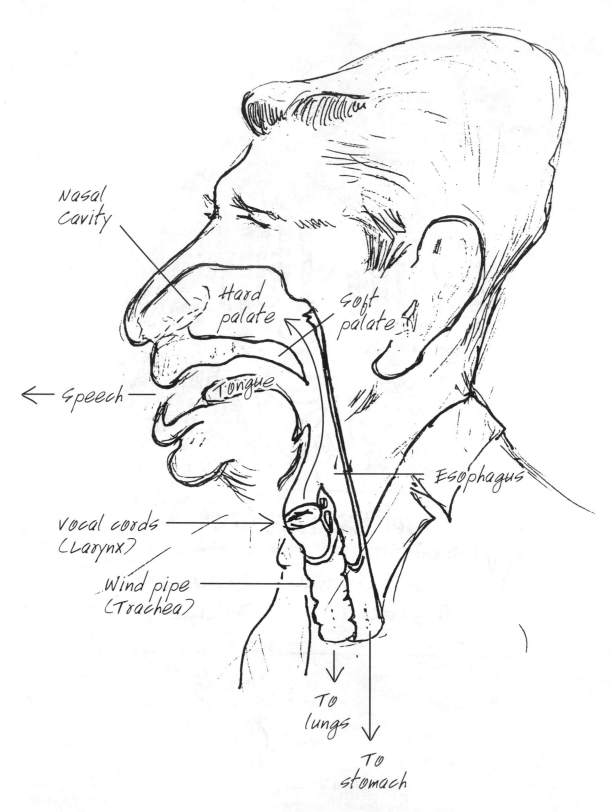

Figure 2–3.

The location of the larynx and other structures of the vocal tract.

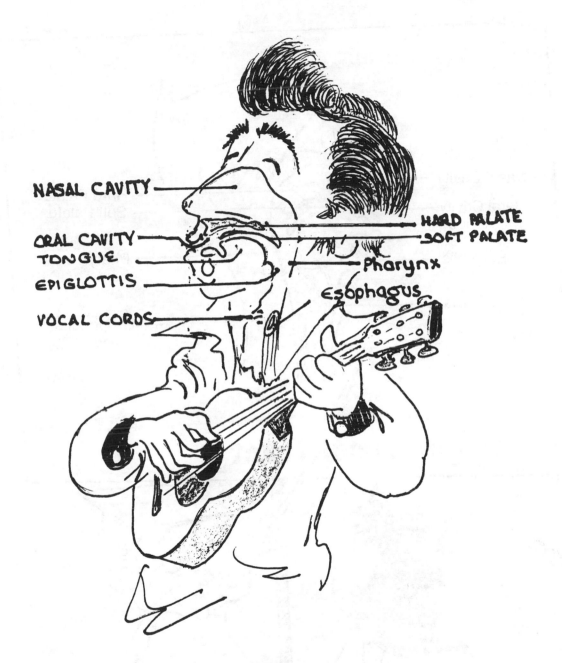

Figure 2–4.
The vocal tract.

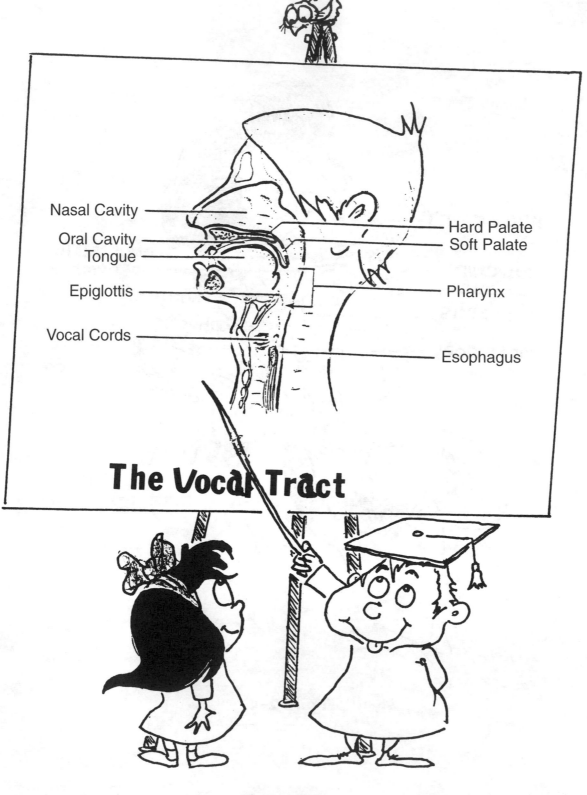

Figure 2–5.
The vocal tract.

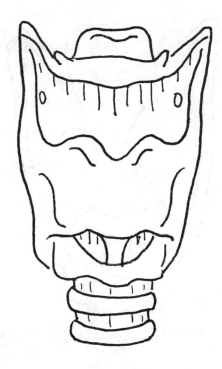

Figure 2–6.
Anterior view of the larynx.

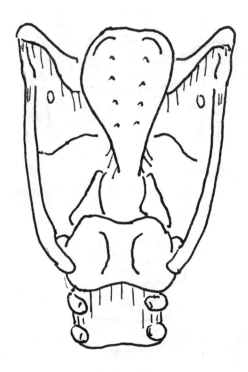

Figure 2–7.
Posterior view of the larynx.

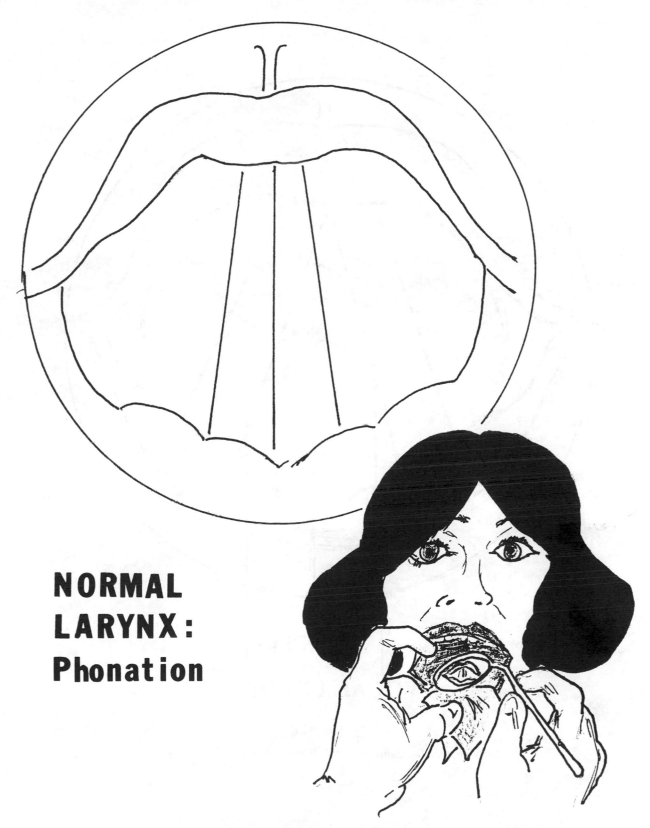

NORMAL LARYNX: Phonation

Figure 2–8.
Mirror examination and superior view of the vocal folds in adducted position.

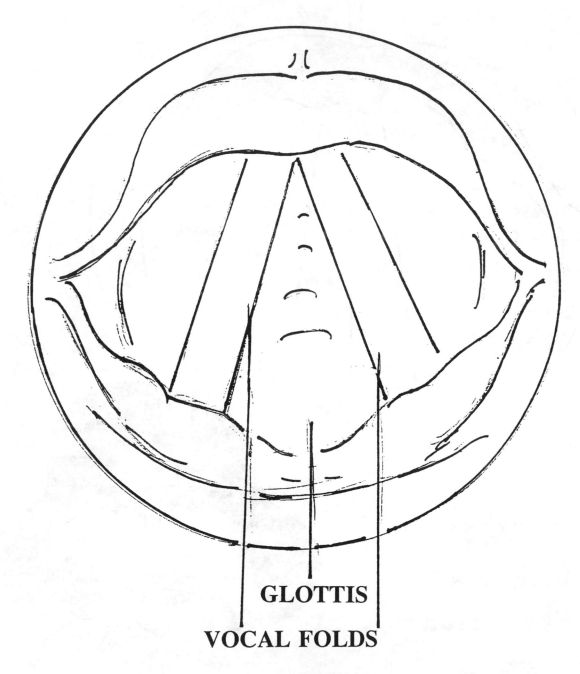

GLOTTIS

VOCAL FOLDS

Figure 2–9.
Superior view of the vocal folds in abducted position.

STAGE

Identify and Label Various Vocal Parameters

Before the group members can learn to discriminate between normal and abnormal voice features, they must be made aware of the various vocal parameters about which they will make judgments. Features such as pitch, loudness, and selected aspects of quality must be identified so that the students may focus their attention on specific parameters of the voice rather than the voice as an undifferentiated whole. Through the activities in Stage III of this program the clinician should attempt to focus the group's attention on the features of pitch and loudness, as well as various aspects of voice quality. The purpose of this stage of the program is to enable the group members to become aware of various vocal parameters that they will be asked to monitor and control in later stages of the program.

GOAL III.A. Group members will be able to identify and vary the vocal parameter of pitch

Procedure III.A.1. Introduce the concept of pitch by using nonvocal sounds

Many students may already have a well developed concept of pitch. Others may have poor or no understanding of pitch. To make the concept as simple as possible we suggest beginning by using sounds other than voice.

Activity III.A.1.a. Many speech-language pathologists have access to a pure-tone audiometer. The audiometer may be used to demonstrate various pitch levels by delivering a signal at high intensity while several students gather close to the earphone. The clinician then simply changes the frequency of the presentation tone, asking the group members to notice these changes.

Activity III.A.1.b. The clinician may use a musical instrument such as a pitch pipe, piano, or harmonica to demonstrate high and low pitch.

Activity III.A.1.c. Students are provided with a list of word pairs and asked which word in each pair is associated with a low pitch and which is associated with a high pitch. For younger children, or for students who have difficulty with the concept of pitch, the clinician may provide a few examples, such as, the cow makes a low pitched sound and the mouse makes a high pitched sound. Suggested pairs are:

foghorn-bell	squeaky wheel-thunder
cat's meow-big dog's bark	flute-tuba
whistle-hum	lion's growl-bird's chirping

This activity may also incorporate drawings or pictures of the items represented in the word pairs. The clinician may wish to use the drawings in Figures 3–1 through 3–14.

Activity III.A.1.d. Ask the group members to provide examples of things that make a high pitched sound and things that make a low pitched sound.

Activity III.A.1.e. Have students solve the word searches at the end of this stage to associate various items/activities with high and low pitch.

Activity III.A.1.f. Have students complete the crossword puzzles at the end of this stage to reinforce the idea that different activities and actions are associated with different pitch levels.

Activity III.A.1.g. Have students solve the scrambled word puzzles at the end of this stage to help develop the concept of pitch.

Procedure III.A.2. Demonstrate variations in vocal pitch

T *Activity III.A.2.a.* Using tape recordings the clinician demonstrates high and low pitch in a human voice.

T *Activity III.A.2.b.* The clinician uses her/his voice to demonstrate high and low pitch by talking at her/his highest and lowest pitch and singing a musical scale.

Activity III.A.2.c. Select members of the group who have different habitual pitch levels and contrast them for the rest of the group.

Procedure III.A.3. Students will vary their pitch

Activity III.A.3.a. Ask each group member to sing up and down the scale as the clinician raises and lowers his/her hand appropriately.

Activity III.A.3.b. Use a drawing of a "pitch ladder" on which students can climb or descend the rungs by raising or lowering pitch while producing a vowel sound (see Figures 3–15 and 3–16).

Activity III.A.3.c. Have each student talk in a high pitch and a low pitch. Avoid extremely high, tense voice production. You may alter this activity (as well as the following activity) by having the group members close their eyes and tapping one on the shoulder to talk in a high or low voice. The other members may then try to guess who is talking.

Activity III.A.3.d. Have the group members read a passage in a "man's voice" then read the same passage in a "woman's voice." For children this activity may be imitation and may use animal characters such as a "lion's voice" and a "mouse's voice."

Activity III.A.3.e. If available, instruments that provide visible feedback regarding pitch such as a Visi-Pitch or Speech Viewer may be used to help students who have difficulty raising and lowering pitch at will.

GOAL III.B. Students will be able to identify and vary the vocal parameter of loudness

Procedure III.B.1. Introduce the concept of loudness by using nonvocal sounds

We would expect that more people would already have a well developed concept of loudness. Therefore, this section probably does not require a great deal of time.

Activity III.B.1.a. As with pitch, a pure-tone audiometer can also be used to demonstrate loudness by adjusting the intensity dial at a given frequency. Increase and decrease the loudness of the signal, pointing out when the signal is loud and when it is soft.

Activity III.B.1.b. A radio or tape recorder may be used to demonstrate differences in loudness by adjusting the volume control.

Activity III.B.1.c. Students are provided with a list of word pairs and are asked which word in each pair is associated with a loud sound and which with a quiet sound. Suggested word pairs are:

motorcycle-bicycle	waterfall-stream
airplane-bird	drum-triangle
motorboat-sailboat	electric guitar-acoustic guitar

Activity III.B.1.d. Students are asked to supply examples of "things that are loud" and "things that are quiet."

Activity III.B.1.e. Use the word searches at the end of this stage to find words associated with soft and loud sounds.

Activity III.B.1.f. Use the crossword puzzles at the end of this stage to reinforce the concept of loud and soft sounds.

Activity III.B.1.g. Have the group members solve the scrambled word puzzles at the end of this stage to further develop the concept of loud and soft sounds.

Procedure III.B.2. Demonstrate variations in vocal loudness

T   *Activity III.B.2.a.* Use tape recorded samples to demonstrate loud and quiet speech. The recordings may be of children, adults, the clinician, or personified animal characters. It is helpful if there is a reference point such as a person speaking normally so that the loud and/or quiet voices can be contrasted with a normal volume.

Activity III.B.2.b. The clinician may demonstrate loud speech and soft speech using his/her own voice. The clinician may talk so low that the group cannot hear him/her or stand close to individual members and speak in a volume that is inappropriately loud.

Activity III.B.2.c. Occasionally a group may include individuals who typically speak louder or more quietly than others. In a manner that would not embarrass the individuals, they may be used as examples of loud and quiet voice. This may sometimes be accomplished by tape recording (or videotaping) a group discussion so that the exemplar members are not conscious of their display status and therefore will speak more naturally.

Activity III.B.2.d. Have the group draw pictures of people talking loudly (someone angry, a cheerleader, a construction worker, etc.).

   Have children draw pictures of people talking softly (mother talking to a baby, a librarian, friends sharing a secret, etc.).

Activity III.B.2.e. Describe attributes of someone with a loud or quiet voice; either physical characteristics (i.e., loud = big person; soft = small, petite person) or personality characteristics (i.e., loud = obnoxious, bossy, peppy; soft = calm, sweet, submissive, shy).

Procedure III.B.3. Students will vary their loudness

Activity III.B.3.a. Ask members of the group to provide examples of their quiet speech. The target here should be a low intensity voice and *not a whisper.* The purpose is to demonstrate that we can all use full voice but it does not have to be loud. Ask group members to provide examples of loud speech. It should be stressed to the group that yelling or screaming is not the target here, but a loud speaking voice. We do not want to encourage vocal abuse, but more important, the purpose is to demonstrate that some "nonyelling" speech can be too loud.

Activity III.B.3.b. Have group members vary their loudness from low to high and high to low. A "loudness ladder" similar to that used in pitch activities may be used to help conceptualize the up and down variations (see Figure 3–17).

Activity III.B.3.c. Instruments that provide visual feedback regarding loudness may be used to help students distinguish loud, normal, and soft voice levels. Computer-based instruments such as the Speech Viewer and the Visi-Pitch are quite helpful if available. Older devices such as the Voice-Lite or the Voice Intensity Controller may be useful. Even devices as simple as the VU meter on a cassette tape recorder may be used to provide feedback regarding loudness.

Activity III.B.3.d. Ask group members questions such as, "Why do we talk quietly?" or "Where do we talk quietly?" Have students generate a list of reasons why we talk softly. Have students generate a list of places where we talk quietly/loudly.

Activity III.B.3.e. Have group members role play speaking situations that require loud or quiet voices. Activities such as telling a secret, talking to a baby or a new kitten, or consoling someone who is grieving can all be used for quiet voices. Talking to a class, speaking to a person with a hearing impairment, or talking over background noise can all be used as examples of loud voice.

GOAL III.C. Students will be able to identify and vary selected aspects of voice quality

Pitch and loudness are relatively easy concepts for most children to understand. Voice quality, however, is a bit more abstract. For purposes of this program, we will limit quality to "Breathy," "Harsh" or "Tense," and "Hoarse." As suggested in some of the following activities, it is often helpful to allow the group members to supply labels for the various voice qualities. Also, because simulating harsh and hoarse voice qualities is more difficult and potentially more abusive than pitch and loudness alterations, this goal incorporates fewer simulation activities.

Procedure III.C.1. Demonstrate various voice qualities

T ***Activity III.C.1.a.*** The clinician can provide examples of breathy, harsh, and hoarse voice quality, pointing out the difference in each example. This may be done with live demonstration or, to reduce the strain on the clinician's voice, an audiotape may be made in which various voice qualities are simulated. It may be helpful for some groups to allow the group members to provide names for these voice qualities. Sometimes student-generated names such as "airy" for a breathy quality or "tight" for a tense or harsh quality are more meaningful to the group. What is important at this stage is that the group members hear the differences in quality and that the clinician and the group members all agree as to which quality a particular label refers.

Activity III.C.1.b. Several commercially available audiotapes, videotapes, and compact disks may be used to provide examples of breathy, harsh, and hoarse voice quality. Examples of such commercially available materials include the CDs that accompany Dworkin and Meleca's (1997) text, or the sound from the video presentation of Stasney (1996).

Procedure III.C.2. Have group members produce a variety of voice qualities

Activity III.C.2.a. Select members to simulate breathy and tense voices. Hoarse voice quality may be difficult for younger children. Be cautious in the simulation of tense and hoarse voice so as not to create an abusive situation.

Activity III.C.2.b. If certain members of the group have distinctive voice qualities they may be used as examples of those qualities. This should be done in a manner that does not embarrass the child selected.

Word Search to Accompany Activity III.A.1.e.

Find the following **high pitch** words:

shriek	woman	creak
peep	child	chirp
meow	whine	squeak
		whistle

```
B E G N O P E E P K

S H R I E K M Q R W

E Q P C R E A K O H

F N T U D Y C E W I

T A C H I L M D G N

C M A J A M L O S E

H O X W H I S T L E

I W A B E H E H N P

R I S Q U E A K S Z

P C V I F C H I L D
```

Word Search to Accompany Activity III.A.1.e.

Answers for **high pitch** words:

shriek	woman	creak
peep	child	chirp
meow	whine	squeak
		whistle

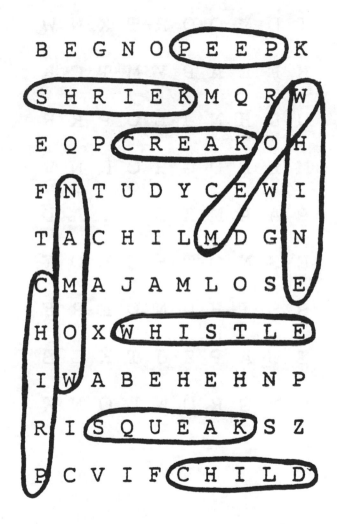

Find the following **low pitch** words:

roar   man   groan
boom   thump   foghorn
moo   growl   thunder

```
A K G T R O A R S J

T D M O O R T X N W

H F E A P Y M T C K

U D H N J L O P R R

M L F O G H O R N V

P A A M X Z B V A D

E S N Q T F E L O Y

S S T H U N D E R F

I U A P Z J T K G B

C N G R O W L O N W
```

Answers for **low pitch** words:

roar   man   groan
boom   thump   foghorn
moo   growl   thunder

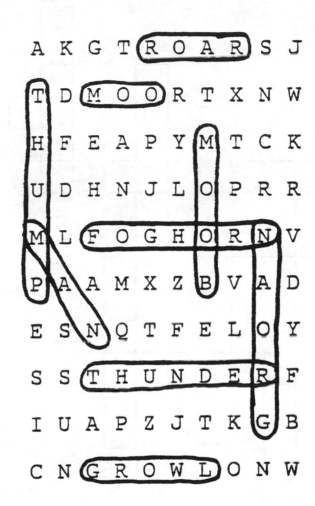

CROSSWORD PUZZLE

High pitch sounds

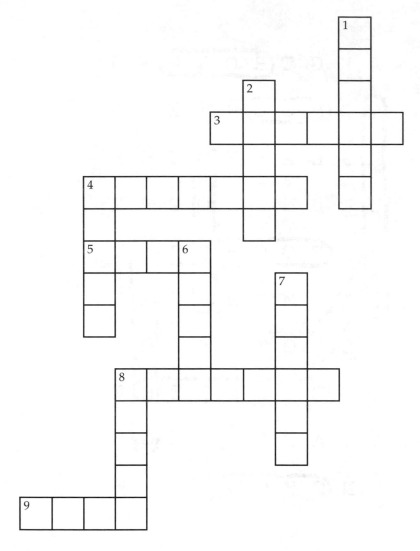

ACROSS:
3. Rhymes with beak _____
4. The seven dwarfs _____ while they work
5. The sound a cat makes _____
8. The floor in the old house _____
9. Don't make a _____

DOWN:
1. Oil the door so it won't _____
2. Man, woman and _____
4. Man has a low voice and a _____ has a high voice
6. _____ and cry
7. The sound a baby pig makes _____
8. The sound a baby bird makes _____

Complete the crossword puzzle using the following words: *chirp, peep, squeak, child, whine, whistle, creaked, meow, woman, shriek, squeal*

CROSSWORD PUZZLE

High pitch sounds

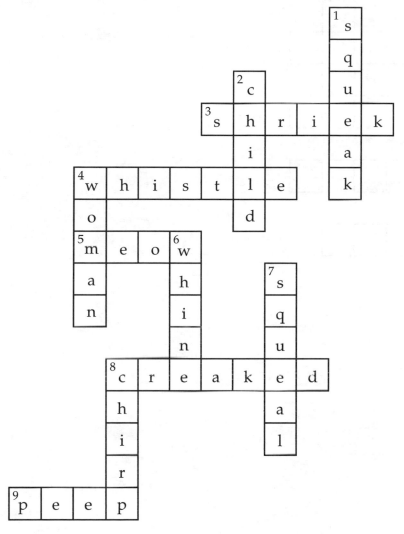

ACROSS:
3. Rhymes with beak _____
4. The seven dwarfs _____ while they work
5. The sound a cat makes _____
8. The floor in the old house _____
9. Don't make a _____

DOWN:
1. Oil the door so it won't _____
2. Man, woman and _____
4. Man has a low voice and a _____ has a high voice
6. _____ and cry
7. The sound a baby pig makes _____
8. The sound a baby bird makes _____

Complete the crossword puzzle using the following words: *chirp, peep, squeak, child, whine, whistle, creaked, meow, woman, shriek, squeal*

CROSSWORD PUZZLE

Low pitch sounds

ACROSS:
3. Sonic _____
4. The ship heard the _____
6. The angry dog _____
7. The crashing _____
8. Woman and _____

DOWN:
1. The tiger let out a fierce _____
2. The sound a cow makes _____
5. When you are in pain you _____
7. The book fell with a loud _____

Complete the crossword puzzle using the following words: *boom, groan, thump, man, foghorn, moo, growled, thunder, roar*

CROSSWORD PUZZLE

Low pitch sounds

```
                    ¹r
        ²m      ³b  o  o  m
         o               a
    ⁴f  o  ⁵g  h  o  r  n
         r
    ⁶g  r  o  w  l  e  d
         a
 ⁷t  h  u  n  d  e  r
  h
  u
 ⁸m  a  n
  p
```

ACROSS:
3. Sonic _____
4. The ship heard the _____
6. The angry dog _____
7. The crashing _____
8. Woman and _____

DOWN:
1. The tiger let out a fierce _____
2. The sound a cow makes _____
5. When you are in pain you _____
7. The book fell with a loud _____

Complete the crossword puzzle using the following words: *boom, groan, thump, man, foghorn, moo, growled, thunder, roar*

53

Scrambled Word Puzzles Associated with Activity III.A.1.g.

Unscramble the following words associated with **low pitch** sounds to find the hidden message. Use the bracketed letters to decode the message.

1. rndetuh   _ [_] _ _ _ _

2. lrgow   _ _ _ [_] _

3. hmput   _ _ _ _ [_]

4. trgnu   _ _ _ _ [_]

5. blumre   _ _ _ _ [_] _

6. mobo   _ [_] _ _

7. wco   [_] _ _

8. igp   _ [_] _

Message: _ _ _ _ _ _ _ _

Solution to **low pitch** scrambled word puzzle.

1. t[h]under

2. gro[w]l

3. thum[p]

4. grun[t]

5. rumb[l]e

6. b[o]om

7. [c]ow

8. p[i]g

Message: <u>l</u> <u>o</u> <u>w</u> <u>p</u> <u>i</u> <u>t</u> <u>c</u> <u>h</u>

Unscramble the following words associated with **high pitch** sounds to find the hidden message. Use the bracketed letters to decode the message.

1. arekc   [_] _ _ _ _

2. ehwni   _ [_] _ _ _

3. dclih   _ [_] _ _ _

4. rasnopo   _ _ [_] _ _ _ _

5. hpicr   _ _ [_] _ _

6. swehlit   _ _ _ _ [_] _ _

7. shis   [_] _ _ _

8. reskih   _ _ _ [_] _ _

9. rigl   [_] _ _ _

Message: _ _ _ _   _ _ _ _ _

56

Solution to **high pitch** scrambled word puzzle.

1. [c]reak

2. w[h]ine

3. c[h]ild

4. so[p]rano

5. ch[i]rp

6. whis[t]le

7. [h]iss

8. shr[i]ek

9. [g]irl

Message: <u>h</u> <u>i</u> <u>g</u> <u>h</u>   <u>p</u> <u>i</u> <u>t</u> <u>c</u> <u>h</u>

Word Searches for Activity III.B.1.e.

Find the following **soft sound** words:

purr   meow   rain
whisper   clicking   squeak
peep   chirp

```
Z  R  R  U  P  I  N  F  M  Q

O  K  S  V  C  L  I  X  D  H

T  C  L  I  C  K  I  N  G  S

S  F  D  E  Y  N  K  R  U  P

C  H  I  R  P  A  V  W  T  E

I  B  P  J  E  N  Q  X  M  E

M  L  W  U  H  G  I  T  J  P

E  B  Q  Z  E  R  D  A  C  K

O  S  T  I  L  N  Q  V  R  S

W  G  W  H  I  S  P  E  R  U
```

Answers for Word Search for Activity III.B.1.e.

Find the following **soft sound** words:

purr	meow	rain
whisper	clicking	squeak
peep	chirp	

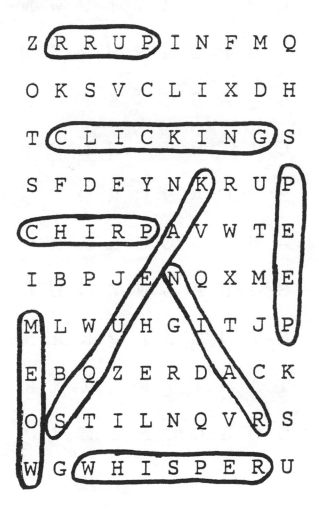

Find the following **loud sound** words:

roar   boom   growl
cry   bang   yell
scream   crash   thunder

G B A C R Y I S W N

I N F U M H M R S T

G Q A S C R E A M F

C I T B V D H L P Y

R W C A N G R O W L

A N B U L C R A K O

S J H A L N Z O H D

H T U G E D P R A K

T A M T Y K I Z X R

D O B O O M G M V J

Find the following **loud sound** words:

roar   boom   growl
cry   bang   yell
scream   crash   thunder

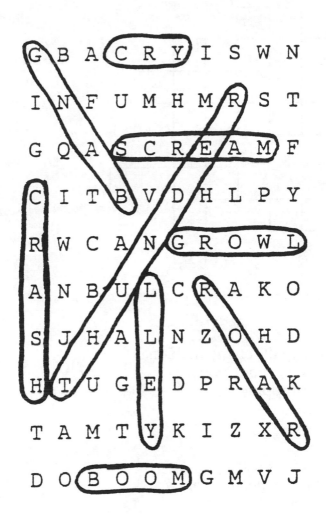

CROSSWORD PUZZLE

Soft sounds

ACROSS:
1. The sound a little bird makes _____
5. The wet _____ softly falls on my umbrella
6. In the library you don't shout, you _____
8. The sound of a pin dropping _____
9. A dog barks, a cat says _____

DOWN:
2. The sound a baby chick makes _____
3. The sound a cat makes when it's happy _____
4. Clocks make this sound _____
7. A mouse makes this sound _____

Complete the crossword puzzle using the following words: *purr, whisper, peep, meow, ticking, chirp, rain, squeak, ping*

CROSSWORD PUZZLE

Soft sounds

Crossword grid:

1 c	h	i	r	2 p		3 p		
				e		u		4 t
				e		5 r	a	i	n
6 w	h	7 i	s	p	e	r		c
		q						k
		u				8 p	i	n	g
	9 m	e	o	w				n
		a						g
		k						

ACROSS:
1. The sound a little bird makes _____
5. The wet _____ softly falls on my umbrella
6. In the library you don't shout, you _____
8. The sound of a pin dropping _____
9. A dog barks, a cat says _____

DOWN:
2. The sound a baby chick makes _____
3. The sound a cat makes when it's happy _____
4. Clocks make this sound _____
7. A mouse makes this sound _____

Complete the crossword puzzle using the following words: *purr, whisper, peep, meow, ticking, chirp, rain, squeak, ping*

63

CROSSWORD PUZZLE

Loud sounds

ACROSS:
4. The two cars made a loud _____
5. The sound a lion makes _____
6. I heard a loud _____
8. An angry dog might _____

DOWN:
1. The scared child will _____
2. Lightning and _____
3. When a baby is hungry he will _____
6. You _____ the drums
7. Please do not _____ at me. I can hear you.

Complete the crossword puzzle using the following words: *cry, bang, scream, roar, boom, growl, yell, crash, thunder*

CROSSWORD PUZZLE

Loud sounds

```
          ┌──┐              ┌──┐
          │¹s│              │²t│
     ┌──┐ ├──┤──┬──┬──┐     ├──┤
     │³c│ │⁴c│ r│ a│ s│     │ h│
┌──┬─┴──┤ ├──┤──┴──┴──┘     ├──┤
│⁵r│ o│ a│ │ r│              │ u│
├──┴──┬─┴──┤ ├──┤           ├──┤
│ y│   │ e│  │ n│
└──┘   ├──┤  ├──┤
       │ a│  │ d│
   ┌──┬┴──┬──┬──┐ │ e│
   │⁶b│ o│ o│ m│ ├──┤
   ├──┤──┴──┴──┤┌─┴──┐│ r│
   │ a│        │⁷y│
   ├──┤        ├──┤
   │ n│        │ e│
   ├──┤──┬──┬──┼──┤
   │⁸g│ r│ o│ w│ l│
   └──┴──┴──┴──┤──┤
              │ l│
              └──┘
```

ACROSS:
4. The two cars made a loud _____
5. The sound a lion makes _____
6. I heard a loud _____
8. An angry dog might _____

DOWN:
1. The scared child will _____
2. Lightning and _____
3. When a baby is hungry he will _____
6. You _____ the drums
7. Please do not _____ at me. I can hear you.

Complete the crossword puzzle using the following words: *cry, bang, scream, roar, boom, growl, yell, crash, thunder*

Scrambled Word Puzzles Associated with Activity III.B.1.g.

Unscramble the following words associated with **soft sounds** to find the hidden message. Use the bracketed letters to decode the message.

1. toonct   _ [_] _ _ _ _

2. rurp   _ [_] _ _

3. ewom   _ _ [_] _

4. alemef   [_] _ _ _ _ _

5. ituqe   _ _ _ _ [_]

6. shiwrep   _ _ _ [_] _ _ _

7. inar   _ _ _ [_]

8. pepdrid   _ _ _ _ _ _ [_]

9. aqusek   [_] _ _ _ _ _

Message: _ _ _ _   _ _ _ _ _

Solution to **soft sound** scrambled word puzzle.

1. c[o]tton

2. p[u]rr

3. me[o]w

4. [f]emale

5. quie[t]

6. whi[s]per

7. rai[n]

8. drippe[d]

9. [s]queak

Message: <u>s</u> <u>o</u> <u>f</u> <u>t</u>   <u>s</u> <u>o</u> <u>u</u> <u>n</u> <u>d</u>

Unscramble the following words associated with **loud sounds** to find the hidden message. Use the bracketed letters to decode the message.

1. tohus   _ _ _ [_] _

2. nutrhed   _ _ _ _ [_] _ _

3. rlgwo   _ _ [_] _ _

4. emsarc   [_] _ _ _ _ _

5. gbna   _ _ [_] _

6. duth   _ _ _ [_]

7. obom   _ [_] _ _

8. elyl   _ _ [_] _

9. tnsuogh   _ [_] _ _ _ _ _

Message: _ _ _ _   _ _ _ _ _

Solution to **loud sound** scrambled word puzzle.

1. sho[u]t

2. thun[d]er

3. gr[o]wl

4. [s]cream

5. ba[n]g

6. thu[d]

7. b[o]om

8. ye[l]l

9. g[u]nshot

Message: <u>l</u> <u>o</u> <u>u</u> <u>d</u>   <u>s</u> <u>o</u> <u>u</u> <u>n</u> <u>d</u>

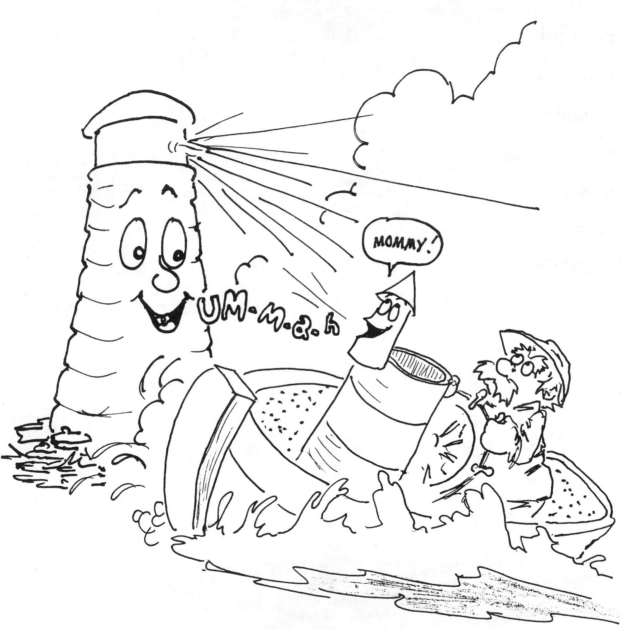

Figure 3–1.
Foghorn.

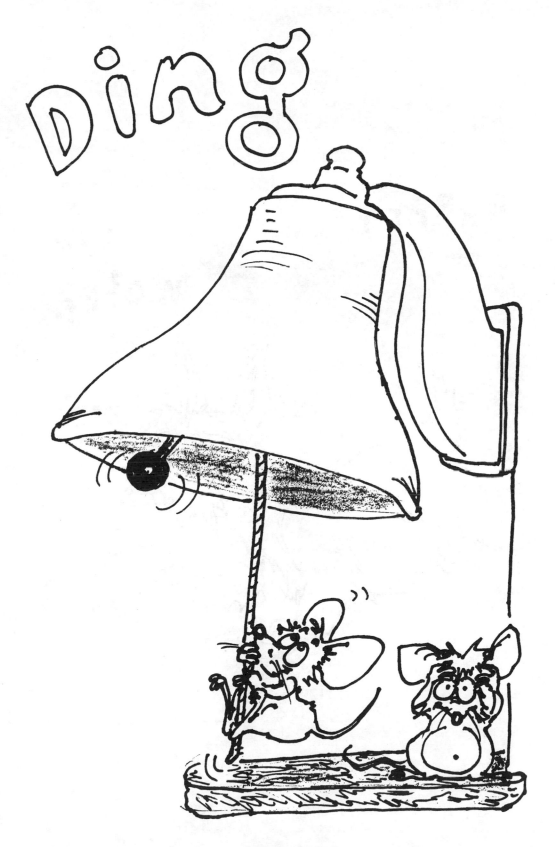

Figure 3–2.
Bell.

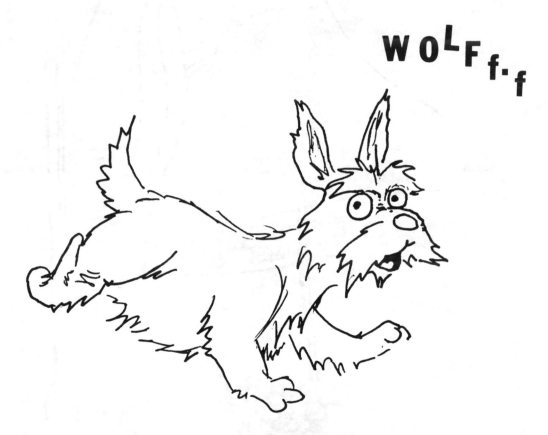

Figure 3–3.
Dog.

MEOW-w-w-w

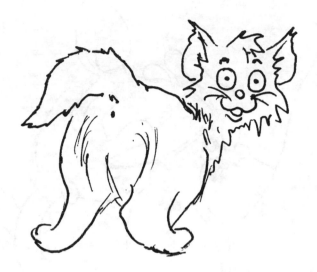

P f f f

Purr-r-r

Figure 3–4.
Cat.

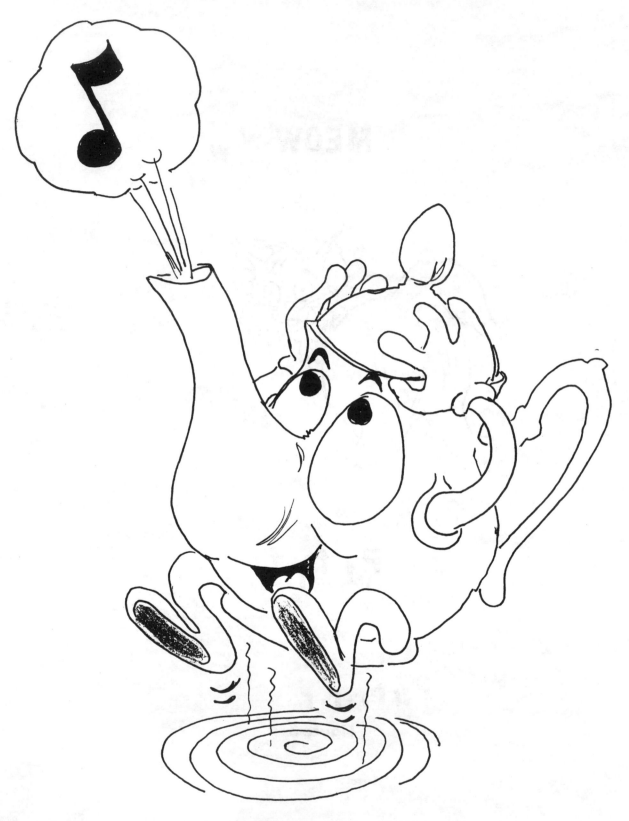

Figure 3–5.
Whistle.

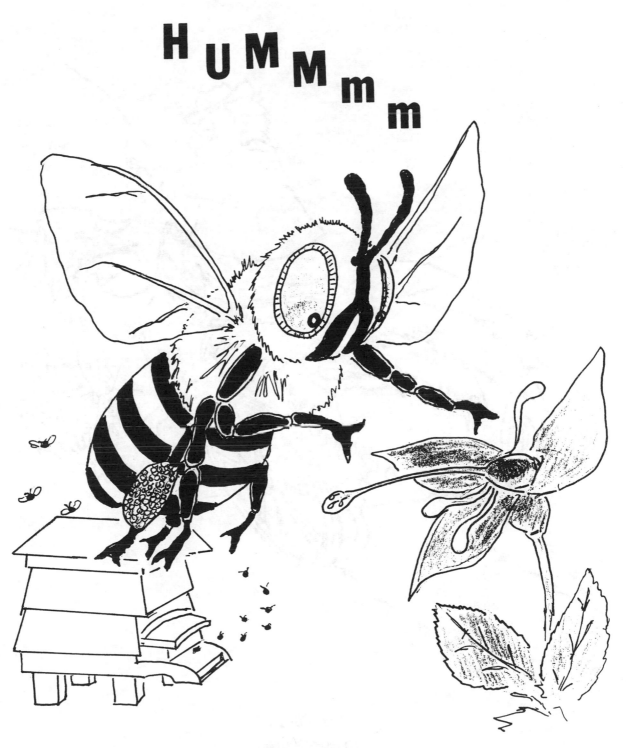

Figure 3–6.
Bee (humming).

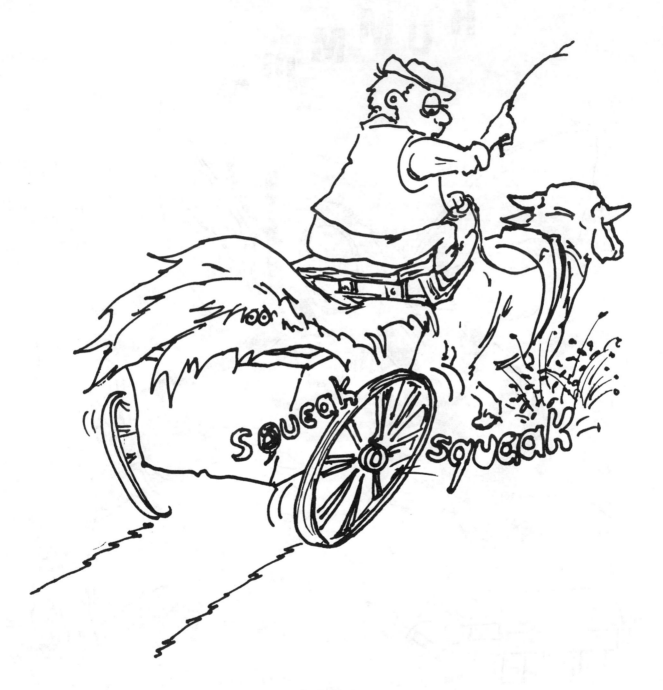

Figure–7.
Squeaky Wheel.

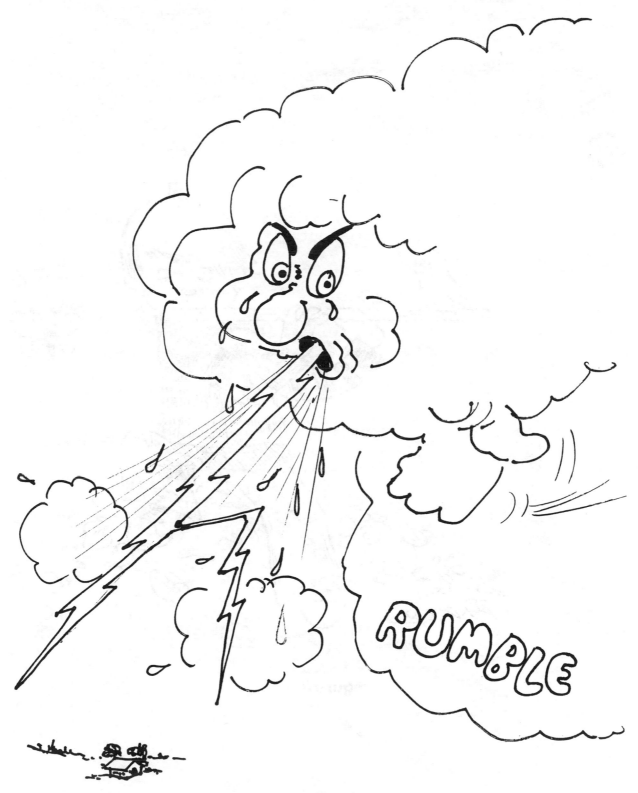

Figure 3-8.
Thunder.

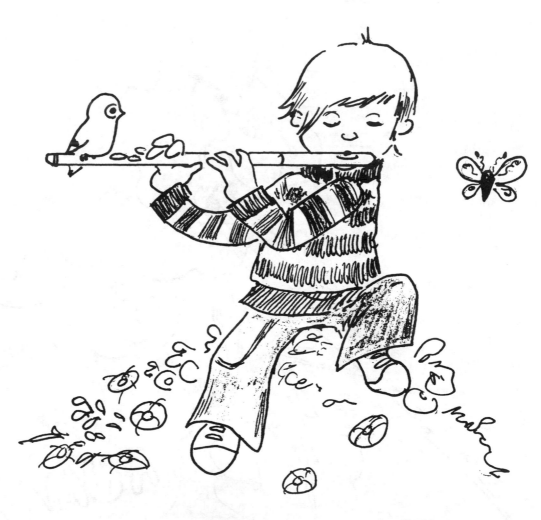

Figure 3–9.
Flute.

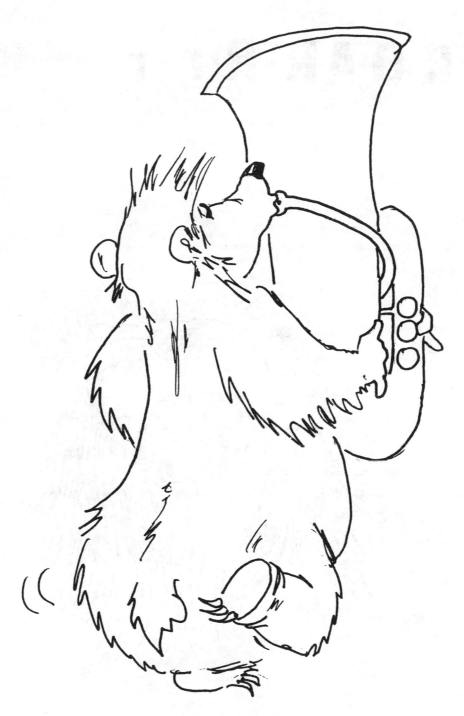

Figure 3–10.
Tuba.

ROAR·R·r·r

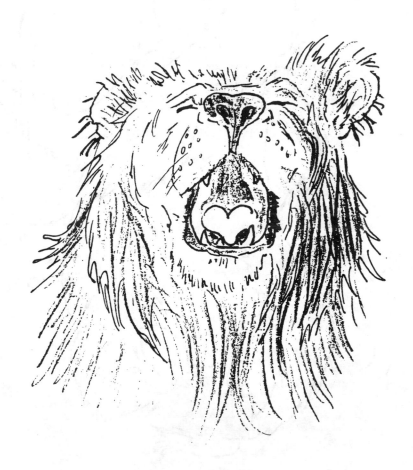

Figure 3–11.
Bear.

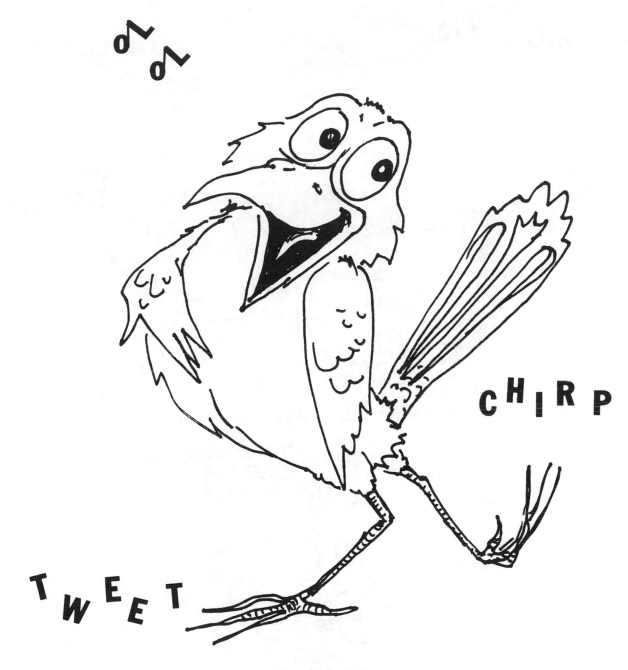

Figure 3–12.
Bird chirping.

MOO·o·o

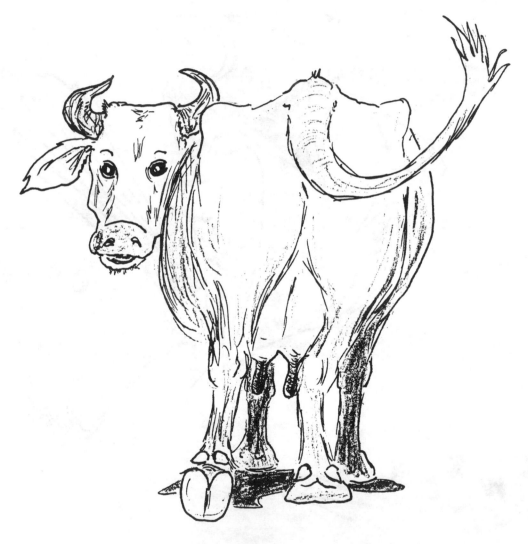

Figure 3–13.
Cow.

ˆsqueakˆ

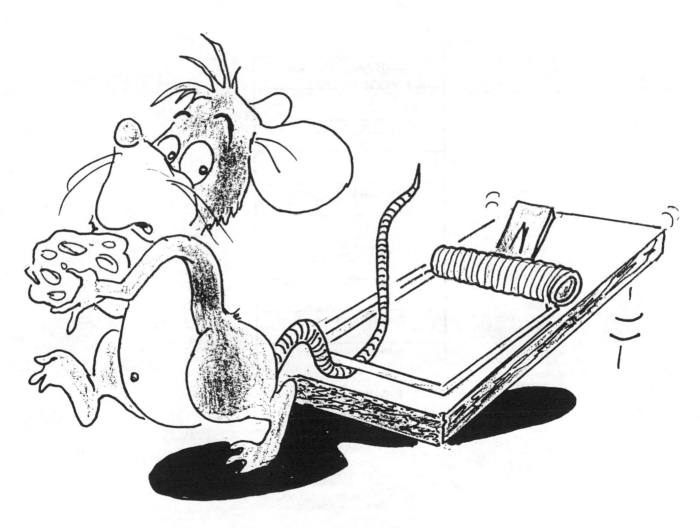

Figure 3–14.
Mouse (squeak).

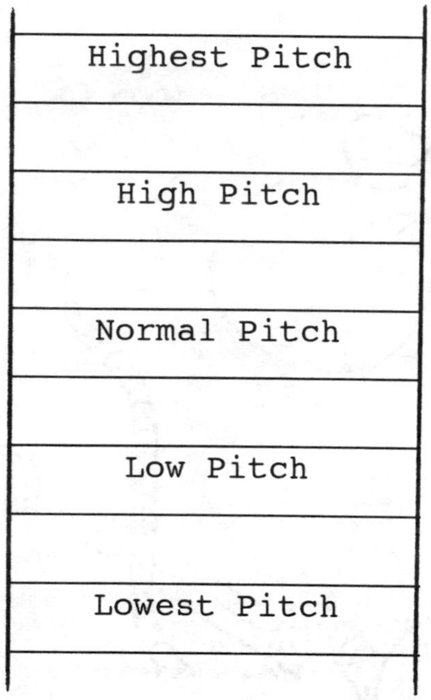

Figure 3–15.
Simple pitch ladder.

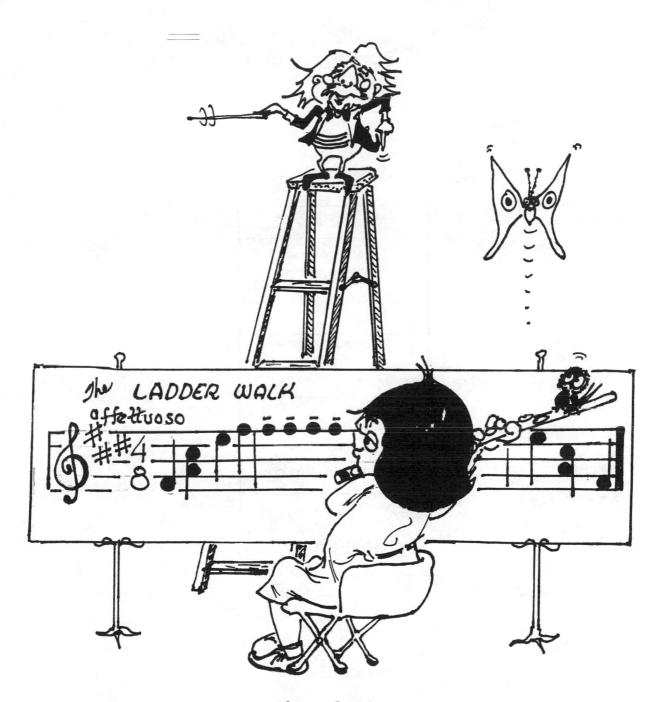

Figure 3–16.
Pitch ladder for older children.

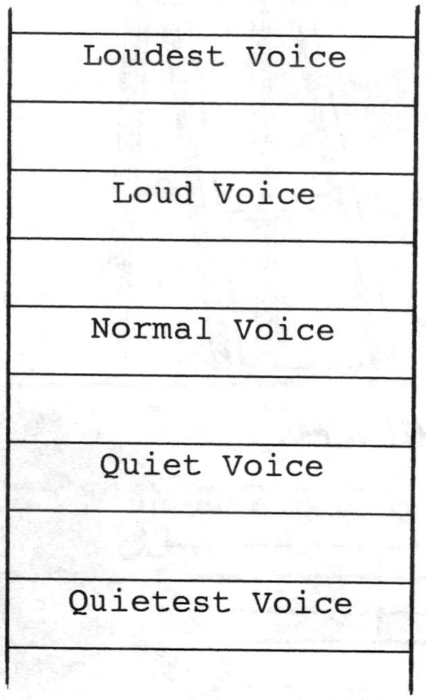

Figure 3–17.
Loudness ladder.

STAGE

Develop Discrimination Skills

Once the group has become familiar with pitch, loudness, and quality, they must learn to distinguish between appropriate and inappropriate displays of these vocal parameters.

GOAL IV.A. Students will distinguish between appropriate and inappropriate pitch

Procedure IV.A.1. Use live voice activities

Activity IV.A.1.a. Speak or read to the group while raising and lowering your pitch to inappropriate levels. Have the students raise their hands when they detect an inappropriate pitch level.

Activity IV.A.1.b. Mark slips of paper with the words (or icons representing the words) high, low, and normal. Have students select the slips of paper from a box. Each student is to speak briefly at the pitch level indicated on the slip. Have the other students indicate whether the speaker is using a pitch that is too high, too low, or appropriate.

Procedure IV.A.2. Using pictures and tape recorded sounds

T P **Activity IV.A.2.a.** Show a picture of a child or a female and play a tape of someone speaking with a low pitch. Ask the students,"What is wrong with this picture?" "What should the pitch of a child or female sound like?" Have the students describe or produce a pitch level that would be appropriate for the picture.

T P **Activity IV.A.2.b.** Show a picture of an adult male and play tapes of a child or a woman speaking with a high pitch. Ask the students, "What is wrong with this picture?" "What should the pitch of a male sound like?" Have the students describe an

87

appropriate pitch (with this age group it will likely be impossible to have group members produce an appropriate pitch to match the picture).

T *Activity IV.A.2.c.* Show a picture of an animal or object and play a tape of a mismatched pitch (i.e., a picture of a mouse paired with the tape of a "moo"; a bell paired with a foghorn). Ask students to talk about what is wrong with the picture. "What should the pitch of the presented picture be?" (Figures 3–1 through 3–14 may be used for this activity.)

T **P** *Activity IV.A.2.d.* Display several pictures of adults (male and female) and children (toddlers through teens). Play tapes of various voices and have the students match pictures to the taped voices. Have them discuss why they matched certain people with certain voices.

T *Activity IV.A.2.e.* Display several pictures of animals or objects and play tapes of the corresponding sounds. Have the students match the pictures to the taped sounds. Have them discuss why they matched certain pictures with certain sounds (use Figures 3–1 through 3–14).

GOAL IV.B. Students will distinguish between appropriate and inappropriate loudness

Procedure IV.B.1. Use live voice activities

Activity IV.B.1.a. Speak or read to the class while increasing and decreasing your loudness. Have the students raise their hands when your loudness level becomes inappropriately loud or soft.

Activity IV.B.1.b. Mark slips of paper with the words (or icons representing the words) loud, soft, and normal. Have students select slips from a box. Each student is to speak briefly at the loudness level indicated on the slip. The other students will indicate if the speaker is using a voice that is loud, soft, or normal.

Procedure IV.B.2. Match pictures of people engaged in various activities with different loudness levels

T **P** *Activity IV.B.2.a.* Show a picture of someone in a quiet setting such as a library, church, or whispering in someone's ear. Play a tape of loud speech and ask, "Is this the right loudness?" Play a tape of a quiet voice and ask "Is this the right loudness?"

T **P** *Activity IV.B.2.b.* Show a picture of someone talking at a normal loudness level such as talking to a group of friends, making a speech, or talking in front of a classroom. Play a tape demonstrating very quiet speech, normal loudness speech, and speech that is too loud. Ask, "Which type of voice is best?" for each presentation. Ask, "Is this the right loudness?"

T P *Activity IV.B.2.c.* Display several pictures of adults and/or children engaged in various speaking activities. Play a tape recorded sample of speech at various loudness levels. Have the students match the pictured activities with the type of voice presented.

Procedure IV.B.3. Discuss appropriate and inappropriate loudness

Activity IV.B.3.a. Lead a discussion about various situations that require a quiet voice and situations in which a speaker may have to use a louder than typical voice.

Activity IV.B.3.b. Have students respond to yes/no questions on a worksheet. The following items are examples of the questions the clinician may use.

	yes	no
Should you shout in a library?	_____	_____
Do cheerleaders talk softly?	_____	_____
Do you scream in church?	_____	_____
Do you yell at your teacher?	_____	_____
Do you whisper in front of a group?	_____	_____

Sentence Completion

Use similar ideas as above, but in sentence completion format.

In a library you should _____.

At a football game the cheerleaders _____.

When talking to your teacher you should never _____ .

When talking to a group you need to talk a little _____.

Procedure IV.B.4. Use taped speech samples

T *Activity IV.B.4.a.* Present various taped speech samples in which people are speaking too loudly, too softly, or at a normal loudness level. Have the group rate each sample as too loud, too soft, or acceptable.

GOAL IV.C. The students will distinguish between abnormal and normal voice qualities

Procedure IV.C.1. Use live voice activities

Activity IV.C.1.a. Speak or read to the class alternately using a breathy, harsh, and hoarse voice quality. Have students identify the quality you exhibit using names they have generated for these qualities (e.g., the "airy" voice for a breathy quality or the "squeezing" voice for a harsh quality).

Activity IV.C.1.b. It is quite difficult for students, especially young students, to provide accurate imitations of various voice quality disorders. However, it is not uncommon for the vocal hygiene group to include members who exhibit an abnormal voice quality, either temporarily or chronically. Select members of the group who exhibit various voice quality deviations. Have these group members speak or read to the rest of the group. The group members are to identify the various voice quality differences exhibited by the speaker.

Note: If this activity is chosen, the clinician must be careful to carry it out in a way that does not embarrass the subjects chosen. In some cases discussing the plan in advance with the chosen group member is all that is needed.

Procedure IV.C.2. Use tape recorded samples

T *Activity IV.C.2.a.* Using a series of tapes, have students identify breathy, harsh, or hoarse voices.

T *Activity IV.C.2.b.* Play tapes of various voice qualities and have students identify what's wrong or different in each voice.

GOAL IV.D. The students will identify inappropriate or inadequate vocal parameters

In the previous activities, the students only had to focus on a single vocal parameter (pitch, loudness, or quality) and were cued as to which parameter would be the focus of their attention. For this goal, students will be asked to listen to voice samples and determine which parameter is inappropriate or inadequate and describe how that vocal parameter is less than acceptable.

Procedure IV.D.1. Use live voice

Activity IV.D.1.a. Speak or read to the group. At various times produce unacceptable pitch, loudness, or quality. Have students raise their hands when they hear an inappropriate or inadequate vocal aspect. Ask them to identify the parameter they felt was not acceptable and in what way it was inappropriate or inadequate.

Procedure IV.D.2. Use taped speech samples

T *Activity IV.D.2.a.* Make a tape recording in which the clinician produces various pitch, loudness, and quality deviations. Play the tape for the students and have them identify the voice deviations. The student responses may be verbal or they may use a prepared voice profile. Several voice profiles are available for use by speech-language pathologists (Boone, 1993; D. K. Wilson, 1987; F. B. Wilson, 1972). The clinician may wish to study these profiles in order to develop one for each particular hygiene group. Voice profiles adapted for use by children are provided in Figures 4–1 and 4–2. On these profiles the children simply have to check one box under each of the three parameters of pitch, loudness and quality.

Activity IV.D.2.b. Make tape recordings or play tapes or CDs of celebrities with unusual vocal pitch, loudness, or quality. Have the students identify and describe the problem vocal parameters. The voice profile in Figure 4–1 and 4–2 may be used for this purpose. Some celebrity voices that might be used include Michael Jackson, Louis Armstrong, Harry Bellafonte, or cartoon characters such as Mickey Mouse or Yosemite Sam.

Activity IV.D.2.c. Use a commercially available tape or CD such as that accompanying the text by Dworkin and Meleca (1997). Follow the same approach as described in **Activity IV.D.2.b.**

Activity IV.D.2.d. Name that voice. Divide the group into teams. Play tapes of various voice qualities and have the teams "Name that Voice." Award points for the correct identification of voice parameters.

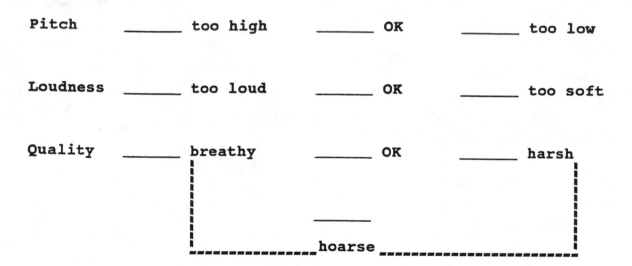

Figure 4-1.

A simple voice profile for children to use.

A voice profile to be used by children in a vocal hygiene group

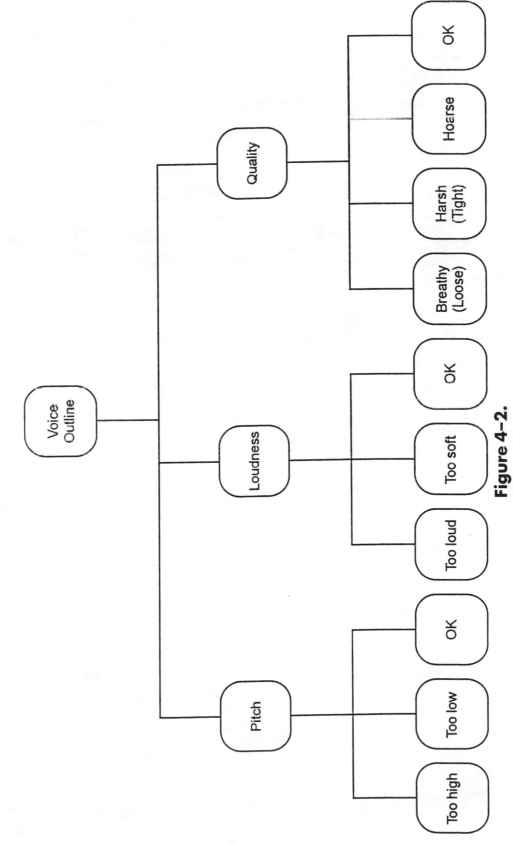

Figure 4–2.

An alternative voice profile for children to use.

STAGE

Identify and Reduce Vocal Abuse

Teaching children that there are certain behaviors that may be harmful to the vocal mechanism and making them aware of alternative behaviors is the essence of any vocal hygiene program. The clinician should be cautious, however, not to make the children fearful of normal vocal activity. We do not wish to create what Sander (1989) referred to as "A population of timid phonophobics-young children who are fearful of loud talking, coughing and perhaps even laughing" (p. 100). Therefore, in this stage of the program the clinician is encouraged to describe the full range of vocally abusive behaviors but to concentrate on reducing or eliminating the most egregiously abusive behaviors.

GOAL V.A. Familiarize students with the nature of vocal abuse

Note: Several authors make a distinction between vocal abuse and vocal misuse. For purposes of this child-oriented program we will not differentiate between these concepts.

Procedure V.A.1. Define and provide specific examples of vocal abuse

Activity V.A.1.a. Simply tell the group, at an appropriate vocabulary level, that vocal abuse is any activity, behavior, or speaking pattern that can injure the vocal folds.

Activity V.A.1.b. Use a vocal abuse checklist to help explain the concept of vocal abuse. Such a checklist allows the clinician to demonstrate the range of activities that can be vocally abusive as well as to help the group focus on the abusive activities in which they engage. Clinicians may make their own checklist, use one from a voice disorders textbook (a very useful one is provided by Case, 1996), or use the accompanying Vocal Abuse Inventory (see Figure 5–1). The Vocal Abuse Inventory presented here is based on lists provided by Case (1996) and by Stemple, Glaze, and Gerdeman (1995). This is not intended to be an all-inclusive list of abuses, simply a starting point to demonstrate the variety of activities and behaviors that may have a deleterious affect on the vocal folds.

Activity V.A.1.c. Make a poster listing the FVI (Federal Voice Inspectors) list of "America's Most Unwanted Voice Enemies." Use the behaviors from the Vocal Abuse Inventory or any other list the clinician may choose (see Figure 5–2).

P   ***Activity V.A.1.d.*** Show pictures of children engaged in vocal abuse activities. Point out to the group the specific behaviors you wish to emphasize and tell them why those behaviors are abusive.

T   ***Activity V.A.1.e.*** Read the following poem to the group, attempting to imitate the various abusive voice qualities of the characters.

Willy Owl's Voice Lesson

Willy was a little owl
who lived out in the wood.
He learned from Uncle Walter owl
the things a young owl should.
Uncle Walter was an older owl
and therefore very wise.
"What will I learn today?" asked Will
with bright and eager eyes.

"Today you'll learn about your voice
and how to keep it strong.
We'll talk of ways to use your voice
and which are right and wrong."
Off they flew to a nearby farm
where Uncle Walter knew
some animals who used their voice
just like some of you.

On their way they came across
Lena the loud loon
who shouted as the owls flew by
in a loud and thundering boom
"Look over here," she said
"Everyone listen to me.
I'm the loudest bird you've ever heard
on the ground or in a tree."

"She sure is loud," said little Willy.
"Is her voice right or wrong?"
"Well if she keeps that up" said Walter,
"She won't have her voice long.
Shouting loud at everyone

doesn't make you a wise bird.
There are better ways my nephew
to be sure that you are heard."

At the farm they soon met Frisky
a gentle little cat
who said, "When friends can't hear me
I move to where they're at.
I never yell, I never scream
I just meow and purr.
That's often a much better way
to let them know I'm there."

In the corn crib was Fast Eddie,
a nervous sort of rat
who, when he talked, he spoke so fast
he sputtered and he spat.
Fast Eddie spoke so rapidly
that it was just plain silly.
"Never try to speak so fast,"
said Uncle Walt to Willy.

Tense Tommy the old turkey
was scratching in the hay.
He was kind of mean and nasty
with nothing nice to say.
His voice was tense and strained
and he used it very hard.
"You owls will have to leave,"
he said, "Get out of my barnyard."

The owls flew out of the turkey's yard
and settled in a tree.
"I've something to say about that voice
so Willy, Listen to me!"
Uncle Walter said, "That grouchy old bird
used a voice with too much force.
A wise young owl won't do that,
if he's smart like you, of course."

They flew next to the barn
where it was warm and dark.
They heard a long deep growl
that was followed by a bark.
Out strode a little puppy
who tried to sound real rough,
"My dad and I are watchdogs
we're the toughest of the tough."

He showed his teeth and growled again
he tried to sound grown-up.
But even though his growl was deep
he still was just a pup.
The owls paid no attention
so the pup just walked away
"To use your voice to sound too tough
is surely not okay."

Once again the birds took off.
"There's one more we must meet.
Just follow me and listen close
then our trip will be complete."
They perched outside the piggies' pen
and heard an awful squeal.
"I'd like to talk, my old friend pig,
if you're finished with your meal."

"We never really finish, Walt
but let's just take a walk.
I grunt and squeal and oink so much
that I can hardly talk.
The noises that we piggies make
are fun and cause a fuss.
But when it comes to talking, pal
It's really hard for us."

"Good-bye my friend," said Walter Owl,
"It's time for us to go.
You've learned a lesson here today
that all smart owls should know.
Recall the sounds the animals made
and listen with a careful ear.
If you use your voice the way they do
it might just disappear."

T *Activity V.A.1.f.* Create a puppet show or plan a skit in which a character with good vocal habits (quiet kitty, gentle gerble, Mrs. Goodvoice, etc.) instructs and points out vocally abusive behavior in a character with abusive vocal habits (loud lion, rough rooster, Mr. Badvoice etc.). A sample script for such a puppet show is presented here.

Sample script for a skit or puppet show to introduce the concept of vocal abuse.

The cast consists of a **narrator** and three puppet characters: **Rough Ralph,** a loud rowdy character with a harsh voice quality, **Shy Sam,** a quiet character who speaks barely above a whisper and tends to keep his head down, and **Melody Goodvoice,** a girl with a pleasant nonabusive voice.

Narrator: "Hi boys and girls! We are here today to talk to you about your voice. We want to show you some things that are good for your voice, and some things that could hurt your voice. I have three friends here to help me today. I'd like for you to meet them. This is Rough Ralph."

Ralph: (In a loud, harsh voice) "Hi kids."

Narrator: "Ralph has a loud voice and sometimes it sounds as though he is really pushing his voice out. Ralph's voice is so loud that it sometimes hurts my ears. Another friend is Shy Sam. Now you have to be very quiet and listen closely because Sam has such a teeny tiny voice it is hard to hear him."

Sam: (In a voice barely above a whisper) "Hi boys and girls."

Narrator: "The last friend I want you to meet is Melody Goodvoice. Melody has such a nice voice that I just love to listen to her."

Melody: (In a clear, gentle voice) "Hello friends, I am happy to be here with you today."

Narrator: "Melody, can you tell Ralph, Sam, and our new friends some things that can hurt your voice?"

Melody: "I'd be happy to. Some of the things that can hurt your voice are:

Screaming and yelling
Talking too loud
Making loud noises when you play with cars or bikes
Making animal or monster noises when you play
Trying to talk in noisy places like when listening to music or on the school bus
Coughing or clearing your throat when you really don't have to."

Ralph: "You mean I can't ever do any of those things?"

Melody: "Sometimes it's OK to do those things, but you should not do them all the time."

Sam: "I don't do any of those things. Does that mean I use my voice correctly?"

Melody: "Well Sam, you might not hurt your voice but you are not using it in the best way that you can. You should talk loud enough so that people can hear you or they won't ever listen to you. What you have to say is important, so don't be afraid to let others hear you."

Narrator: "Thank you Melody. Now let's see what we have learned. Ralph, would you count to five for us please."

Ralph: (In a loud, harsh voice) "1,2,3,4,5."

Narrator: (Asking the group members) "Boys and girls, was that a good voice?"

(Hopefully the response will be "No.")

Narrator: "Ralph, try that again in your best voice."

Ralph: (Now in an acceptable loudness and quality) "1,2,3,4,5."

Narrator: "Very good Ralph, you've learned a lot. Sam, would you count to five for us?"

Sam: (In a voice barely above a whisper) "1,2,3,4,5."

Ralph: "Did he say it? I couldn't hear him."

Narrator: "Remember Sam we all want to hear you. You don't have to yell but don't be afraid to let your voice do its job."

Sam: (In an acceptable loudness and quality) "1,2,3,4,5."

Narrator: "Did you hear him boys and girls?" (Response,"Yes") "Very good Sam. Let's see how Sam and Ralph can use what they've learned at school."

New scene, at school, Sam sits alone with head down. Enter Melody.

Melody: "Sam, What's wrong? You look so sad."

Sam: (In his weak voice) "I am sad because when I talk people don't listen and I don't have any friends."

Melody: "Well I'm your friend, Sam, and I can help you. Remember what you learned about letting your voice do its job? Look at people when you talk to them, take a good breath before you begin to talk and let your voice come out."

Sam: (at first in a weak voice) "OK, first I look at you, then I take a good breath (now in a strong but not loud voice), and then let my voice come out. What I have to say is important!"

Melody: "Oh, Sam that sounds so much better."

Ralph: (From off-stage in his loud, harsh voice) "Vroom Vroom I can't wait until I can drive a car."

Melody: "I can hear Ralph coming before I can see him."

Melody and Sam: (Covering their ears) "His voice hurts our ears."

Ralph: (loud voice) "Hi guys, What are you doing?"

Melody: "Ralph, you are using your loud voice and I heard you making car noises."

Ralph: (In an acceptable loudness) "I'm sorry I forgot. I can talk softer but I do like to play cars, what can I do?"

Sam: "When I play cars, I make noise with my lips like this (bilabial raspberry). That doesn't hurt my voice at all."

Melody: "Good idea, I think you boys are learning how to use your voice."

Narrator: "Well Sam and Ralph learned a lot about their voice. Let's see what you've learned."

Tell me some things that can hurt your voice.
Should you never, ever do any of these things?
What should you do if your voice is too loud?
What should you do if your voice is too weak?

Activity V.A.1.g. Have students complete the crossword puzzles with words describing good vocal behaviors and vocally abusive behaviors.

Activity V.A.1.h. Assign the word search activity at the end of the section.

Activity V.A.1.i. Assign the scrambled word puzzle at the end of this stage.

Activity V.A.1.j. Hangman: divide the students in groups of two or more and play hangman, using vocabulary words dealing with those at risk for voice problems (i.e., shouting, coughing, cheerleading, etc.).

Activity V.A.1.k. Divide the group into two or more teams to play Vocal Abuse Pictionary. A member of one team is given a form of vocal abuse. That person attempts to draw a picture that will allow his or her team to guess which form of abuse he or she is attempting to represent. Encourage the team to make as many guesses as possible so that they will be thinking of all of the various forms of abuse.

Procedure V.A.2. Identify situations that contribute to vocal abuse

Activity V.A.2.a. Explain to the group that certain situations lend themselves to vocal abuse and people must be careful not to overwork their voice in these situations. Such situations include:

athletic contests (spectator)	talking to large groups
athletic contests (participant)	playgrounds
noisy places	swimming pools
noisy equipment	riding bikes

Activity V.A.2.b. Have students generate a list of people who are at risk for developing voice problems due to their job, hobbies, activities, and so on.

Activity V.A.2.c. Present a list of people/situations to the group. Have the students identify which are most likely to abuse their voice. Such a list may include:

Cheerleader	Coach
Librarian	Rock singer
P.E. teacher	Someone who whistles a lot
The loudest student at school	Someone who argues a lot
People who talk over loud noise	A singer who follows the singing teacher's advice
Someone who claps loudly at ball games	A singer who does not follow the singing teacher's advice
	Boys and girls who make car and motorcycle noises when they ride bikes

GOAL V.B. Identify vocal abuse in others

Procedure V.B.1. Identify vocal abuse from photos and drawings

P *Activity V.B.1.a.* Show pictures of children engaged in activities that suggest quiet vocal activity (talking softly to a pet, whispering in someone's ear, reading, etc.) and pictures of children exhibiting vocally abusive behaviors (yelling at a sporting event) and have the group identify the vocally abusive activity.

Activity V.B.1.b. Have each member of the group draw a picture showing someone doing something that is vocally abusive and something not abusive. Show the pictures to the rest of the class and have them select the abusive and nonabusive behaviors.

Activity V.B.1.c. Using a chalkboard, poster, or feltboard, write out various vocal behaviors that are abusive and some nonabusive vocal behaviors and/or nonvocal behaviors such as clapping for your favorite team, whistling to call your dog, and so on. Have the children place, write, or instruct you to place each activity in the appropriate category. The categories could be abusive versus nonabusive, healthy voice use versus hurtful voice use, voice friendly versus voice unfriendly, or any terms the clinician feels appropriate for the group.

Procedure V.B.2. Identify vocal abuse from audio and videotapes

Activity V.B.2.a. Play audiotapes or CDs of rock singers known for their abusive singing styles (e.g. Janice Joplin, Joe Cocker) and of singers with smoother styles (Mel Torme, Bing Crosby) and ask the group to indicate which singer is showing vocal abuse.

Activity V.B.2.b. Play a video or audiotape of television shows such as Sesame Street in which some of the characters have abusive voice patterns (Cookie Monster, Beaker the lab assistant) and others do not. Have the children indicate which characters are exhibiting vocal abuse.

T *Activity V.B.2.c.* Videotape or audiotape the group or another group of children at play. Have the group identify the vocally abusive behaviors exhibited in the tape.

T *Activity V.B.2.d.* Videotape or audiotape a role playing activity in which adults or children purposely exhibit vocally abusive behaviors. Have the group members identify as many of the target behaviors as they can.

GOAL V.C. Identify the vocal abuse patterns of group members

Procedure V.C.1. Group members identify activities they engage in that may be vocally abusive

Activity V.C.1.a. Use the Vocal Abuse Inventory introduced in **Activity V.A.1.b.** as a checklist which the group members may complete as a profile of their personal vocal abuse patterns. Group members should be encouraged to add any activities they think are abusive.

Activity V.C.1.b. Ask each member of the group to carry a small spiral notebook and write down each time they engage in a vocally abusive activity between this session and the next meeting of the group. Begin the next meeting by reviewing the books of each member.

Procedure V.C.2. Have others help to identify the vocally abusive behaviors of group members

Activity V.C.2.a. Involve parents, siblings, or teachers as "abuse monitors." Send a note to those parents, siblings, or teachers who might be willing to help. Instruct them to ask the child if a particular behavior might be vocally abusive when they hear the child engage in such behaviors.

Activity V.C.2.b. Divide the group into pairs who will act as "voice monitors" for each other. The voice monitor will point out vocal abuse to his or her partner. Instances of disagreement may be brought to the clinician or the group at a later meeting for a judgment.

Activity V.C.2.c. Tape record the children during a "free" activity or play period. The clinician, with the help of other group members, should listen for and identify instances of vocal abuse by the group members.

GOAL V.D. Students/clinician will suggest alternatives and modifications to vocally abusive behaviors

Procedure V.D.1. The clinician will provide specific suggestions for alternative behaviors to and modifications of vocally abusive behaviors

Activity V.D.1.a. The clinician will provide a generic list of suggestions for substitute behaviors and modifications of abusive behaviors. That list may include any or all of the following:

1. Walk closer to people instead of yelling to them.
2. Whistle or clap hands rather than yell to attract attention, call pets, or cheer on your team.
3. Bring a shaker to a game and shake it rather than yell.
4. Signal with flashlights or by turning the house lights on and off rather than calling from one room to another.
5. Use your natural pitch. Do not try to speak at a lower or higher pitch level to try to create a desired effect.
6. Avoid grunting during strenuous exercise such as weight lifting or aerobics (This behavior has even become common among female tennis players). Try substituting a forceful burst of air.
7. Develop your listening skills so that you do not always dominate conversations (Boone, 1991).
8. Try to move away from background noise before talking.
9. Be sure to have the attention of your listener.
10. Try a hard swallow rather than clearing your throat.
11. Try a "voiceless" cough rather than throat clearing.
12. Consult a physician and be sure to follow his/her instructions with regard to medication to reduce coughing and allergy symptoms.
13. Sing quietly, hum, or whistle rather than singing loudly over music or in the shower.
14. Drink more water and fruit juice instead of coffee, tea, and cola drinks.

For older clients:

15. Use amplification when talking to groups.

16. If you smoke and cannot quit, allow yourself to smoke only outside in some other specific location. The more inconvenient the location, the better.

Procedure V.D.2. Have group members generate suggestions for alternate behaviors or modifications

Activity V.D.2.a. Ask each group member to suggest activities that he or she could substitute for the vocally abusive behaviors he or she exhibits.

Activity V.D.2.b. Select group members who will describe their specific abuses and entertain suggestions from the rest of the group for alternatives or modifications.

Activity V.D.2.c. Describe a situation or read a short story in which someone is using a vocally abusive behavior. Ask the group to suggest alternatives for the abusive activity. The stories that follow may be used for this purpose or serve as examples of stories which may be created by the clinician.

Story #1

John was taking his dog Buster for a walk in the park. As they were walking Buster stopped and looked in the direction of a small pile of leaves. There was a rustling sound coming from the pile. Just then a small gray squirrel stuck his head out of the pile, saw John and Buster, and took off running across the park. Buster immediately began chasing the squirrel. The dog ran off so quickly that he yanked his leash right out of John's hand. John began to yell as loud as he could, "Buster! Buster come back. Buster get back here you crazy dog!"

What is John doing that could hurt his voice? (Yelling for his dog.)
What could he do instead? (Whistle, clap, have Buster fetch a stick and return it to John, shake a box of doggie treats to tempt Buster to return.)

Story #2

Lashon and his friends are at a football game. The game is very close and the cheerleaders are telling the crowd, "Make some noise!" Lashon and his friends scream and yell as loud as anybody in the stands. After the game, Lashon finds that his voice is hoarse and it hurts a bit to talk.

Why do you think Lashon is having problems with his voice? (He has been yelling too loud and too long.)
What could he have done at the game that would have helped his voice stay strong? (Whistle, stomp, clap, use a noisemaker, etc.)

Story #3

Rosa and Maria are at a school dance. They are standing near the front of the gym where the speakers are located. The music is very loud. They like to sing and talk. But in order to be heard above the music they must be very loud.

What are Rosa and Maria doing that could harm their voice? (Talking and singing over loud background noise.)
What are some things that they could do to help their voice? (Move away from the speakers. Try to talk between songs.)

Story #4

Keiko has a cold and a very bad cough. Every time she coughs or clears her throat she can feel her throat becoming more and more sore. Her voice is getting worse and worse. She tries not to cough but sometimes she just can't help it.

What is Keiko doing that is damaging her voice? (Coughing and clearing her throat.)
Is there anything that poor Keiko can do to reduce her coughing and make her throat less sore? (See her doctor and follow his advice. Be sure she takes any medicine that the doctor or her parents think will help. Drink plenty of fluids.)

Story #5

Frank and Antonio went to the State Fair on a Saturday afternoon. The fair was very crowded. Frank became separated from Antonio and began to look for his friend. After a few minutes Frank spotted Antonio at the cotton candy stand. Frank yelled to Antonio but the crowd was so noisy that Antonio could not hear his friend. Frank yelled louder and made the "Wildcat Roar" (an animal noise used at their school at pep rallies and games) to try to attract Antonio's attention.

What is Frank doing that could harm his voice? (Yelling and making a loud animal noise.)
What are some things that Frank could do instead of yelling for Antonio? (Run over to Antonio. Whistle, wave, etc.)

Story #6

Every year Melissa enjoys Christmas caroling with her friends. She also likes to sing in the school choir and at the parties she attends at this time of year. The parties are fun and she sings and laughs and talks over the music playing. This year she notices that after caroling in the neighborhood for about an hour her voice is becoming a bit hoarse and her throat a bit scratchy. Melissa does not want to go home and leave her friends because they are having so much fun.

Why might Melissa's voice be getting hoarse? (Using her voice too much by singing and partying.)
What can she do tonight and for the rest of the Christmas season to help her voice? (Tonight she could just tag along with the group and not sing. For the rest of the season she should reduce the amount of singing and loud talking at parties.)

Story #7

Mother is putting dinner on the table. Mark is watching television while his brother Kevin is upstairs doing homework. Mother asks Mark to tell Kevin that dinner is ready and the boys should wash their hands and come to the table. Mark, without moving from his chair, yells as loud as he can, "Kevin, dinner is ready. Wash your hands." Mark yelled so loud that the family's pet cat, Nervous Nellie, leaped from the back of the chair where she was sleeping and hid under the sofa.

What did Mark do that could harm his voice? (Yelled for his brother.)
What could Mark have done that would have been better for his voice? (Walked upstairs to tell his brother that dinner was ready, flashed the upstairs lights as a signal that Kevin was to come downstairs, rang a bell to summon his brother, etc.)

T   *Activity V.D.2.d.*   Present a puppet show or a skit in which a character is abusing his or her voice. Have another character ask the group members to help provide some alternative behaviors to help the abusing character reduce his or her vocal abuse. The characters described in **Activity V.A.1.f.** may be used here with a script similar to this:

Melody:	"Ralph, you aren't talking as loud or yelling as much as you used to, but there are still some times when I hear you using your voice in a hurtful way."
Ralph:	"I know, Melody, but sometimes it's hard not to yell. Is there anything I can do instead of yelling at a football game?"
Narrator:	"Well, Ralph, maybe we can ask our friends. Boys and girls what can Ralph do instead of yelling at a football game?" (Try to elicit responses such as clap, whistle, use a noise maker if they are allowed, etc.)
Ralph:	"Thanks, those are good ideas. But what can I do instead of yelling for my pet dog Rover?"
Narrator:	"Boys and girls?" (Encourage responses such as whistle, clap, etc.)
Ralph:	"How about when the other kids are playing with bikes and cars, do I just have to be quiet?"
Narrator:	"Well, let's hear what our friends have to suggest." (Encourage suggestions such as lip sounds (raspberries) or buccal sounds, etc.)

GOAL V.E. Begin to reduce abuse in a systematic manner

Procedure V.E.1. Establish a baseline of abusive behaviors

Activity V.E.1.a. Provide group members with a small spiralbound note pad that contains a list of abuses identified earlier. Each person is to record each time he/she exhibits that abuse.

Activity V.E.1.b. Have group members audiotape or videotape speaking activities in which they are engaged (presentations, concerts, phone conversations, athletic events, etc.) and count the number of abuses during those activities.

Procedure V.E.2. Target specific behaviors to be reduced

Activity V.E.2.a. Have each member of the group select one of the abuses identified in **Procedure V.E.1.** as his or her "target" behavior. Discuss with each member how he or she plans to reduce this behavior. The clinician should provide suggestions and guide the children in making certain that each plan is realistic.

Activity V.E.2.b. The clinician may examine the data collected in **Procedure V.E.1.** and select for each child what appears to be their most frequent or most abusive behavior, or the behavior which appears to be the easiest to eliminate. The selected behavior will then become the "target" behavior for each child.

Procedure V.E.3. Involve others in the abuse reduction activities

Activity V.E.3.a. Involve parents and teachers in the monitoring of target behaviors. One way to do this is to simply inform the parents or teachers about the target behavior and ask them to help remind the child whenever they hear the behavior.

Activity V.E.3.b. Have each child complete a request for assistance form similar to the one provided in Figure 5–3 to be given to parents, teachers, coaches, or other adults who are involved in activities with the children. The form can be completed by inserting the child's name and the target behavior in the appropriate blank space.

Activity V.E.3.c. Have the students chart their instances of vocal abuse. Because the actual instructional program will likely not continue long enough to monitor these behaviors for very long, the charting begun here should also continue as a carry-over activity and will be mentioned again in Stage VI. Charts may be as simple or as complex as the clinician feels the group can handle. But as a rule, in order to enhance the chances of the children doing this, the simpler the better. An example of a simple chart is provided in Figure 5–4.

Activity V.E.3.d. Have parents (or teachers) designate an article of clothing, selected accessories, a piece of jewelry, and so on as a "good voice reminder." This technique is similar to tying a string around one's finger to remember to do something. The very presence of the object serves as a reminder. For example, a parent could provide the child with an inexpensive ring, a pair of different colored shoelaces, a hair ribbon, or a ball cap and indicate that this item is to remind the child to avoid the targeted abusive behavior.

Activity V.E.3.e. Use a token economy to reward the reduction of the targeted abusive behavior. At the beginning of each day, parents (or a teacher) can provide the child with a number of objects (paper clips, pennies, plastic tokens, slips of paper, etc.) Each time the parent (or teacher) hears the child exhibit the targeted abusive behavior, the child must surrender one of the objects. At the end of a specified time (day, week, etc.) the child will be allowed to redeem the objects for some treat. The more objects he or she is able to keep, the more valuable the treat he or she can select.

Activity V.E.3.f. Have the children make a contract with the clinician, a teacher, or parents to reduce at least one form of vocal abuse. Such a contract may be modeled after the one in Figure 5–5.

CROSSWORD PUZZLE

Good Voice Words

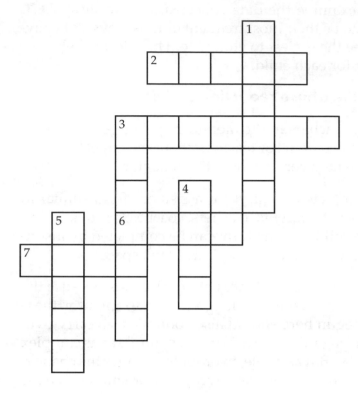

ACROSS:
2. A library is this kind of place
3. _____ instead of yell
6. Take it _____ and easy
7. _____ your hands when happy

DOWN:
1. The opposite of rough _____
3. Tell me a secret
4. The opposite of hard _____
5. Let me make it _____

Complete the crossword puzzle using the following words: *clap, clear, gentle, quiet, slow, soft, whisper, whistle*

CROSSWORD PUZZLE

Good Voice Words

ACROSS:
2. A library is this kind of place
3. _____ instead of yell
6. Take it _____ and easy
7. _____ your hands when happy

DOWN:
1. The opposite of rough _____
3. Tell me a secret
4. The opposite of hard _____
5. Let me make it _____

Complete the crossword puzzle using the following words: *clap, clear, gentle, quiet, slow, soft, whisper, whistle*

CROSSWORD PUZZLE

Vocal Abuse Words

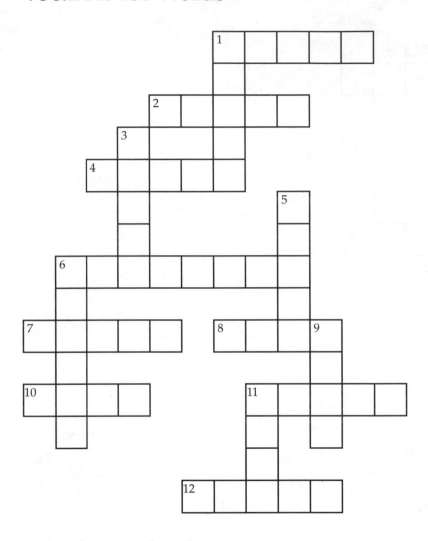

ACROSS:
1. Don't _____ like a tiger
2. Use a silent _____ to clear your throat
4. Whistle, don't _____ to your friend
6. If you talk too much your voice will become _____
7. Don't moan and _____
8. Whistle, don't _____ for your pet
10. Slow down, don't talk too _____
11. His voice was _____ like sandpaper
12. Don't use such _____ words

DOWN:
1. The sound a grown pig makes _____
3. Clap, but don't _____ at the game
5. Don't _____ in Switzerland
6. If you see a spider don't _____
9. Hush, don't talk so _____
11. A lion sound

Complete the crossword puzzle using the following words: *cheer, cough, groan, growl, grunt, harsh, loud, roar, rough, scream, shout, strained, yell, yodel*

CROSSWORD PUZZLE

Vocal Abuse Words

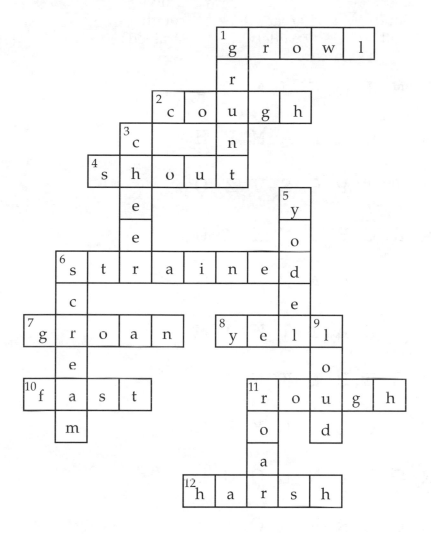

ACROSS:
1. Don't _____ like a tiger
2. Use a silent _____ to clear your throat
4. Whistle, don't _____ to your friend
6. If you talk too much your voice will become _____
7. Don't moan and _____
8. Whistle, don't _____ for your pet
10. Slow down, don't talk too _____
11. His voice was _____ like sandpaper
12. Don't use such _____ words

DOWN:
1. The sound a grown pig makes _____
3. Clap, but don't _____ at the game
5. Don't _____ in Switzerland
6. If you see a spider don't _____
9. Hush, don't talk so _____
11. A lion sound

Complete the crossword puzzle using the following words: *cheer, cough, groan, growl, grunt, harsh, loud, roar, rough, scream, shout, strained, yell, yodel*

111

Word Searches for Activity V.A.1.h.

Find the following words associated with vocal abuse:

cheer	cough	fast	groan	growl
grunt	harsh	loud	roar	rough
scream	shout	yell	yodel	strained

```
A  Z  N  T  O  F  J  N  X  S

L  N  S  C  R  E  A  M  P  H

H  H  I  T  P  O  S  V  Z  O

G  A  R  G  R  U  N  T  K  U

U  R  L  G  O  A  F  A  S  T

O  S  L  H  A  T  I  W  A  M

C  H  E  E  R  B  K  N  T  L

D  T  Y  O  D  E  L  X  E  U

G  R  O  W  L  N  L  O  U  D

H  G  U  O  R  E  H  Q  K  Y
```

Answers for Word Searches for Activity V.A.1.h.

Find the following words associated with vocal abuse:

cheer   cough   fast   groan   growl
grunt   harsh   loud   roar   rough
scream   shout   yell   yodel   strained

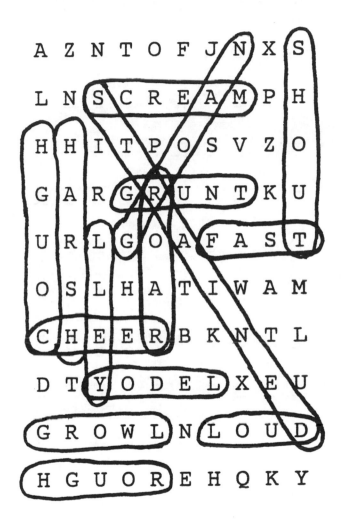

Find the following words associated with a good voice:

clear   gentle   clapping
quiet   slow   whistle
soft   whisper

```
E P C L I Y G B D R

S L O W P T E Z H T

O W I V X D N F G V

F D H F R K T A N H

T S U I A N L O I R

Q W H I S P E R P S

B E H W C T K X P D

L Y G E N W L J A Q

G E B Z F R A E L C

A Q U I E T J M C U
```

Answers to Word Search

Find the following words associated with a good voice:

clear   gentle   clapping
quiet   slow   whistle
soft   whisper

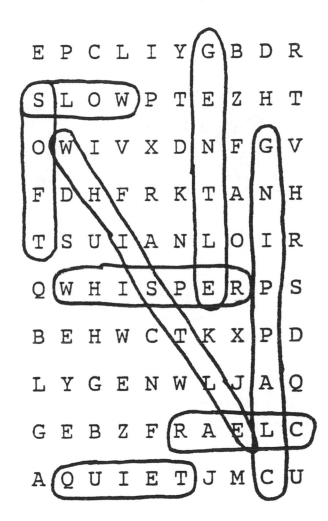

E P C L I Y G B D R
S L O W P T E Z H T
O W I V X D N F G V
F D H F R K T A N H
T S U I A N L O I R
Q W H I S P E R P S
B E H W C T K X P D
L Y G E N W L J A Q
G E B Z F R A E L C
A Q U I E T J M C U

Unscramble the following words associated with vocal abuse to find the hidden message. Use bracketed letters to decode the message.

1. omeulv   [_] _ _ _ _ _

2. gohur   _ _ [_] _ _

3. uchog   _ [_] _ _ _

4. ehere   [_] _ _ _ _

5. casmre   _ _ _ _ [_] _

6. putarb   _ [_] _ _ _ _

7. hutos   [_] _ _ _ _

8. lyel   _ [_] _ _

9. hsrha   _ [_] _ _ _

10. deylo   _ _ _ _ [_]

Message: _ _ _ _ _   _ _ _ _ _

KEY: Word Scramble for words associated with vocal abuse.

1. [v]olume

2. ro[u]gh

3. c[o]ugh

4. [c]heer

5. scre[a]m

6. a[b]rupt

7. [s]hout

8. y[e]ll

9. h[a]rsh

10. yode[l]

Message: <u>v</u> <u>o</u> <u>c</u> <u>a</u> <u>l</u> <u>a</u> <u>b</u> <u>u</u> <u>s</u> <u>e</u>

Vocal Abuse Checklist for Children

How often do you do each of these?	never	occasionally	frequently
yelling on the playground			
yelling while playing sports			
cheering at sporting events or pep rallies			
cheerleading			
loud talking			
making animal noises			
making motorcycle or car or truck noises			
any other unusual noises made with voice			
talking at a high or low pitch			
singing in an abusive manner			
talking in noisy places			
participation in plays and other speaking or singing performances			
calling pets			
yelling to other people			
calling loudly for family members at home			
verbal arguments with friends or siblings			
any other yelling or screaming			
talking for long periods of time			
loud laughing			
coughing			
throat clearing			
smoking			

Figure 5–1.

A vocal abuse inventory.

Federal Voice Inspectors (FVI)

10 most unwanted voice behaviors

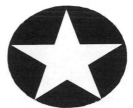

- 1. Screaming
- 2. Talking too loud
- 3. Making monster/animal noises
- 4. Making car noises (motor or tire squealing
- 5. Using a pitch that is too high
- 6. Using a pitch that is too low
- 7. Talking in noisy places
- 8. Throat clearing
- 9. Coughing
- 10. Making any sounds that make your throat hurt

Figure 5–2.
Most Unwanted Vocal Behaviors.

Help Me To Keep My Voice Healthy

Dear _____

    I am currently enrolled in a voice education program at school. An important part of this program is to help me reduce or eliminate behaviors that can be damaging to my voice. The activity that I am trying to reduce is _____.
It would be very helpful if you could remind me about my voice every time you hear me_____.
All you need to do to remind me is to point at me or even look at me in a meaningful way. Thank you for helping me to keep my voice healthy.

_____

Student

_____

Speech-Language Pathologist

Figure 5–3.
Request for assistance in monitoring vocal abuse.

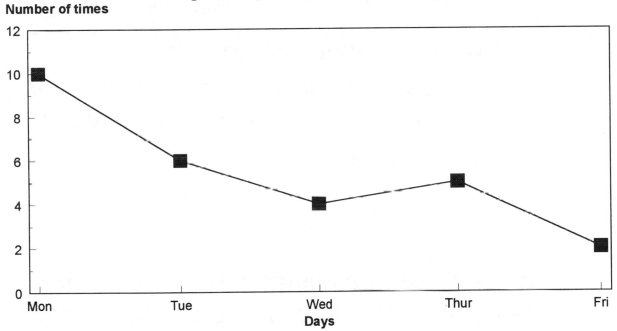

Figure 5-4.

An example of a simple vocal abuse reduction chart.

Good Voice Contract

▼

- This contract is made between
  _____ a student
  learning about voice and

  _____

  the parent/teacher of the student.
- The student promises to reduce or eliminate
  the following vocally abusive behaviors:

  _____

  _____

  _____

- If the student eliminates or reduces the
  behaviors listed above he/she will receive

  _____

- Signatures

  _____   _____

  student   parent/teacher

Figure 5–5.
Contract to reduce vocal abuse.

122

STAGE

Summarize and Facilitate Carryover

A vocal hygiene program typically offers a great deal of information over a predetermined number of sessions. For the program to have a lasting effect on the participants, it should include some activities designed to summarize the information presented and to facilitate transfer of that information to "out-of-class" situations. Through the activities in this final stage of the program, we hope to maximize the effect of the program on the children who took part.

GOAL VI.A. Reiterate important points from the program

Procedure VI.A.1. Clinician reviews major points

Activity VI.A.1.a. Simply provide a review of the most important points of the program. This review should stress those aspects of the program that the clinician emphasized during the previous sessions. In almost all cases, it would be expected that the awareness and reduction of vocal abuse would be stressed in such a review.

Activity VI.A.1.b. Use the outline of the program presented in Section I. of this manual as a guide for constructing a review.

Procedure VI.A.2. Review material by quizzing the class

Activity VI.A.2.a. Use the following list of questions to form the basis of a review. The clinician may select the questions he/she feels best represent the program as it was presented. The clinician may also add questions to the list. The questions may be presented in oral or written form and may be addressed to the group or to selected individuals.

1. What do we call the structure that we use to produce voice?

2. Where is that structure located? (Students may point or provide a description such as, "In the neck" or "On top of the trachea" depending on the level of sophistication of the group.)

3. What do we call the muscles that vibrate to make voice?

4. Is this sound a high pitched or a low pitched sound? (Clinician makes a high pitched sound.)

5. Is this sound a high pitched or a low pitched sound? (Clinician makes a low pitched sound)

6. Is this a good way to use your voice or a bad way? Why? (Clinician speaks in an excessively loud voice or plays a tape of someone speaking in an excessively loud voice.)

7. Is this a good way to use your voice or a bad way? (Clinician makes loud car noise or animal noise or plays a tape of such sounds.)

8. Name some things that people do that are bad for their voice.
OR
Which of these activities can harm your voice?

   ❖ yelling at a football game
   ❖ talking quietly
   ❖ making loud noises when playing cars or riding bikes
   ❖ making loud animal noises when playing or reading
   ❖ humming quietly
   ❖ clearing your throat a lot
   ❖ singing real loud
   ❖ singing gently
   ❖ yelling to pets or to other children

9. What can people do instead of the harmful voice activities identified in Question 8?
OR
For each of the activities you said were harmful to your voice in Question 8, suggest a substitute activity that would not be harmful.

10. What are the three most important things you learned in this class?

   ❖ This question often provides some surprising answers. The students' answers can sometimes be very rewarding to the clinician or sometimes frustrating.

GOAL VI.B. Provide tangible reminders regarding appropriate and inappropriate voice usage

Procedure VI.B.1. Make use of a student notebook

Activity VI.B.1.a. Boone (1991) provided a list of "Ten easy steps for keeping your voice natural." Boone's list, which follows, may be provided to older groups or adapted to the age and maturity of each group:

1. Cut down on throat clearing and coughing; don't yell
2. Develop an easy voice attack
3. Use a pitch level that is natural for you
4. Develop good vertical and horizontal focus for your voice
5. Renew your breath more often by pausing
6. Reduce demands on your voice; don't do all the talking
7. Develop an open vocal tract
8. Avoid talking in loud settings
9. Avoid smoking and excessive use of alcohol (with populations under 21 delete "excessive")
10. Watch your water needs: humidity and liquids

Activity VI.B.1.b. Create a list of do's and don'ts. An example of the types of items that might be included in such a list may be found in Table 6–1. The list should be provided to each member of the group.

Activity VI.B.1.c. Use Figure 6–1 through Figure 6–13 to illustrate vocal do's and don'ts. These figures may be placed into students' notebooks, colored in or used in any other way that the clinician feels would be appropriate.

Activity VI.B.1.d. Have each group member make a personal list of vocal behaviors that he or she agrees to continue to monitor and reduce after completion of the program.

Activity VI.B.1.e. Wilson (1987) described voice treatment plans for children which incorporated a 10-step outline. He was able to apply the same 10 steps to reduce, eliminate, or modify various target voice behaviors. Such a 10-step outline could be incorporated into a vocal hygiene program as a final checklist for abusive behaviors targeted for reduction by individual group members. An example of a 10-step outline from Wilson (1987) is presented below. This particular outline addresses shouting, but it should be clear to the clinician how easily a variety of vocal behaviors could be targeted:

1. I know the rule about not shouting.
2. I can tell when other people shout.
3. I can tell when other people are not shouting.
4. I know how my voice sounds and feels when I shout.
5. I know how my voice sounds and feels when I don't shout.
6. I know the places where I usually shout.

7. I know the places where I don't shout.

8. I can keep from shouting some of the time.

9. I can keep from shouting most of the time.

10. I don't shout anymore.

Such a list could be placed in each group member's notebook. The stages already achieved could be checked off by the clinician and the student could have the completion of the checklist assigned as a carryover activity. A parent or teacher would check off the last step at some time after the completion of the program.

Procedure VI.B.2. Develop a contract

Activity VI.B.2.a. Use a list such as that described in **Activity VI.B.1.b.** but place that list in the content of a formal agreement between the clinician and the group member. The agreement could be similar to that described in **Activity V.E.3.f.**

Activity VI.B.2.b. If a contract was developed in Stage V of this program, that contract may be extended to cover one or more additional abusive behaviors.

GOAL VI.C. Reward the group members for completing the program

Procedure VI.C.1. Provide mementos of completion

Activity VI.C.1.a. Provide each member of the group with a certificate of completion. Examples of such certificates are found in Figures 6–14 and 6–15.

Activity VI.C.1.b. Have the group make and color cardboard buttons to be pinned or taped to their clothing indicating that they completed the program.

Activity VI.C.1.c. Provide each group member with a ribbon on which something is written indicating the completion of a vocal education program.

Procedure VI.C.2. Use activities to mark the completion of the program

Activity VI.C.2.a. Have a "good voice party." This can be a pizza or ice cream party in which the group members are reminded to use their voice in an appropriate manner. Games and activities should be selected that do not encourage loud voice use such as charades.

Activity VI.C.2.b. Take the group on a field trip to a place where they must use a quiet voice. Such places as a theater, concert, or museum might be appropriate.

Voice DO'S and DON'TS

- DO
- Reduce coughing and throat clearing
- Use shakers and noisemakers at games
- Use a pitch level that is natural for you
- Renew your breath more often by pausing
- Drink lots of water
- Move close enough to people to be heard without yelling

- DON'T
- Yell or scream
- Talk in noisy places
- Always do all the talking
- Make loud car animal or monster noises when playing
- Call for pets or people over long distances
- Sing at pitch or loudness levels that are uncomfortable
- Talk too fast

Table 6–1.
A list of vocal do's and don'ts.

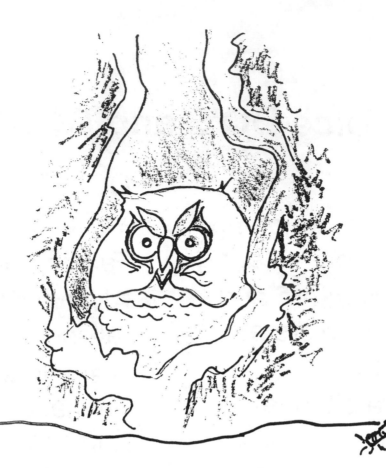

BE WISE

DO NOT

MAKE
↑ANIMAL OR MACHINE NOISES

TALK TOO LOUD

SCREAM OR YELL

TALK TOO HIGH OR TOO LOW

COUGH LOUD OR TOO MUCH

Figures 6–1 through 6–13.
These figures are all self-explanatory reminders to reduce or eliminate various forms of vocal abuse.

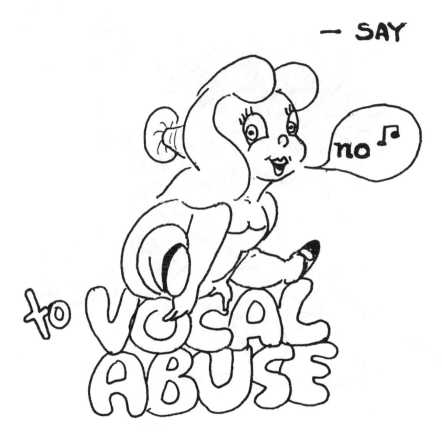

Figure 6-2.

Relax

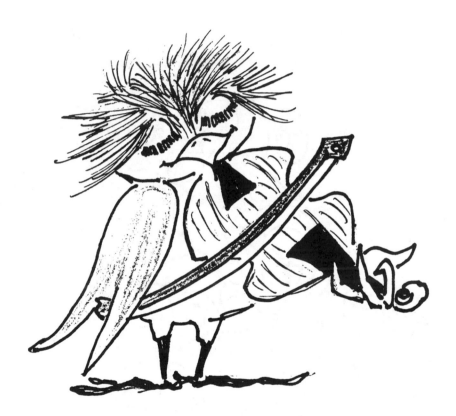

your

Voice

Figure 6–3.

S p e a k

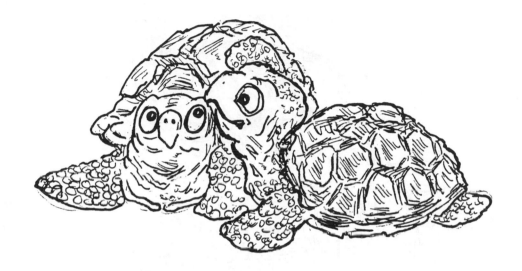

S · L · O · W

a n d

e a s y

Figure 6–4.

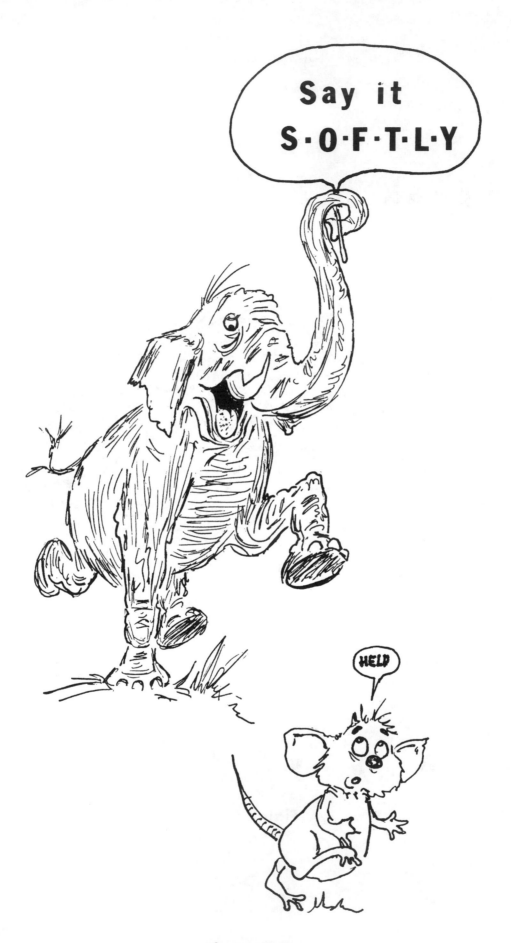

Figure 6–5.

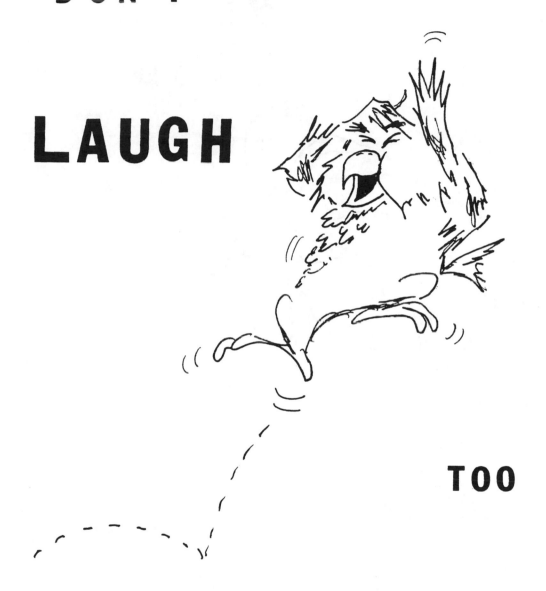

DON'T

LAUGH

TOO

LOUDLY

Figure 6–6.

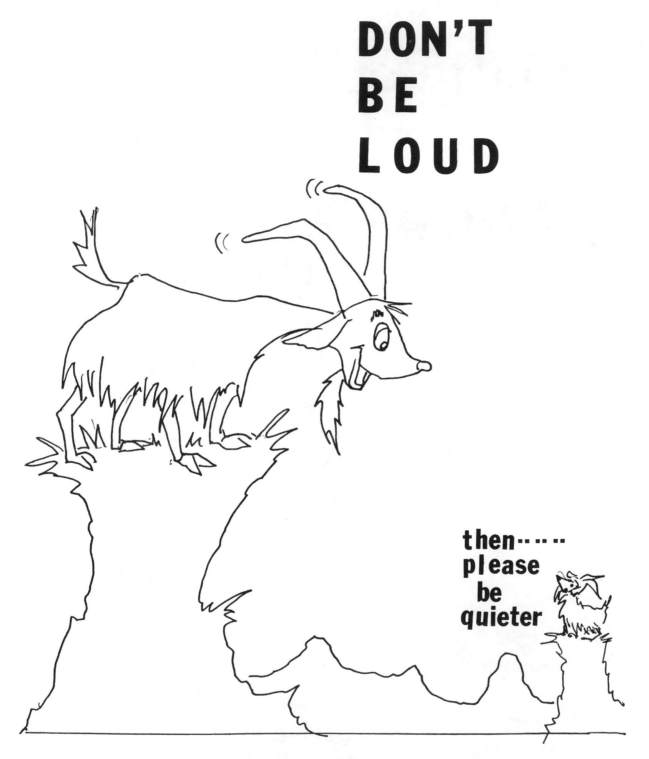

Figure 6–7.

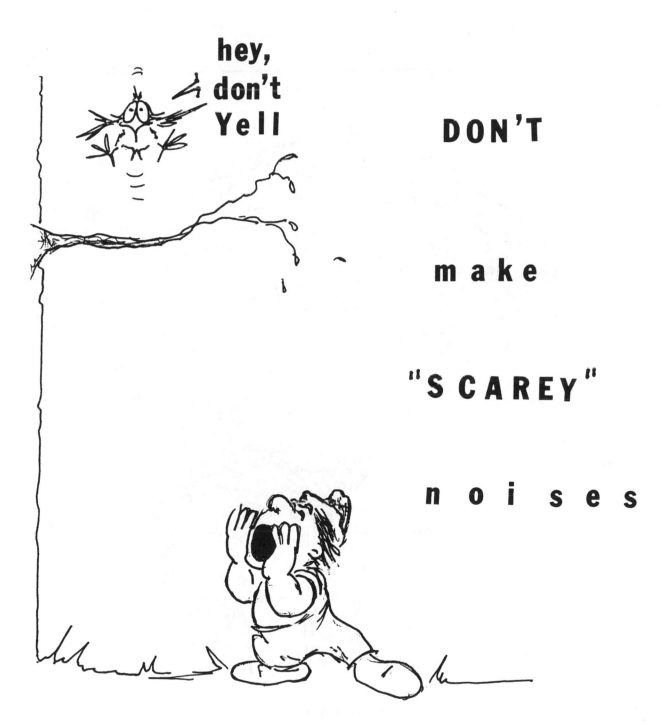

Figure 6-8.

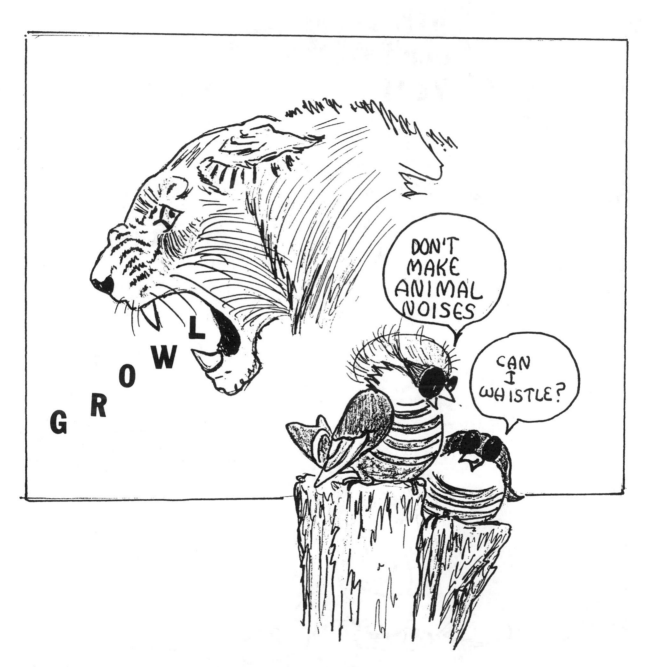

Figure 6–9.

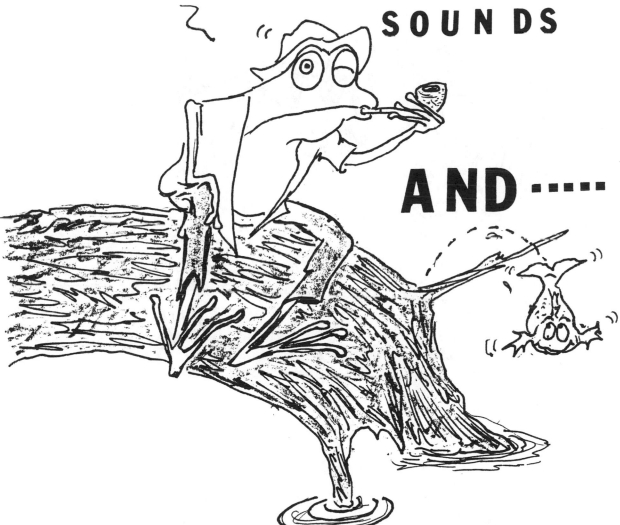

Figure 6-10.

137

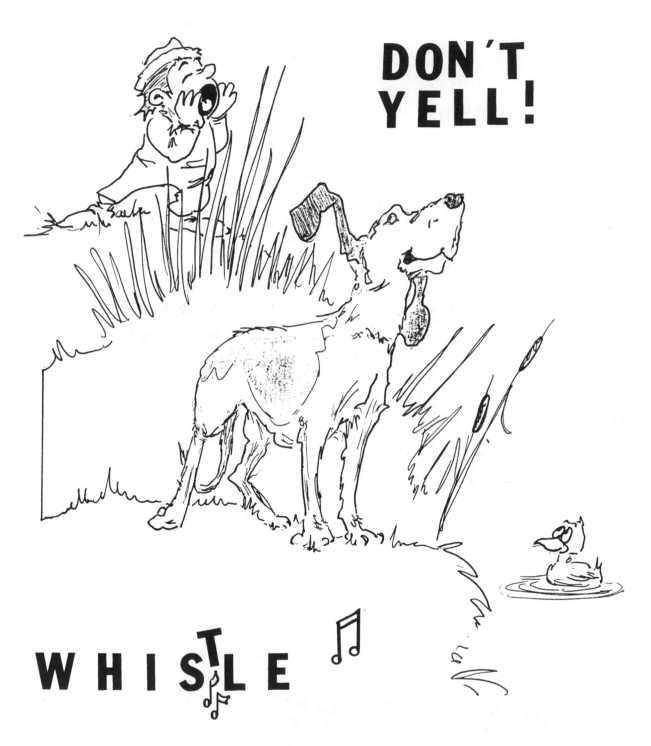

Figure 6-11.

HOW

QUIET

AM

I

?

I

LOVE

GENTLE

VOICES

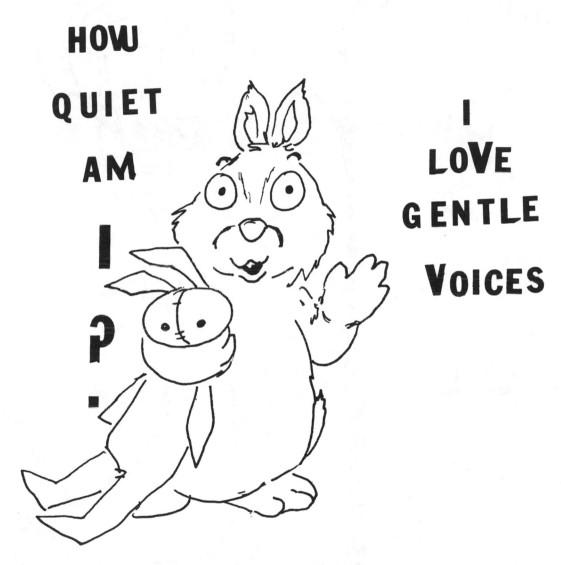

Figure 6-12.

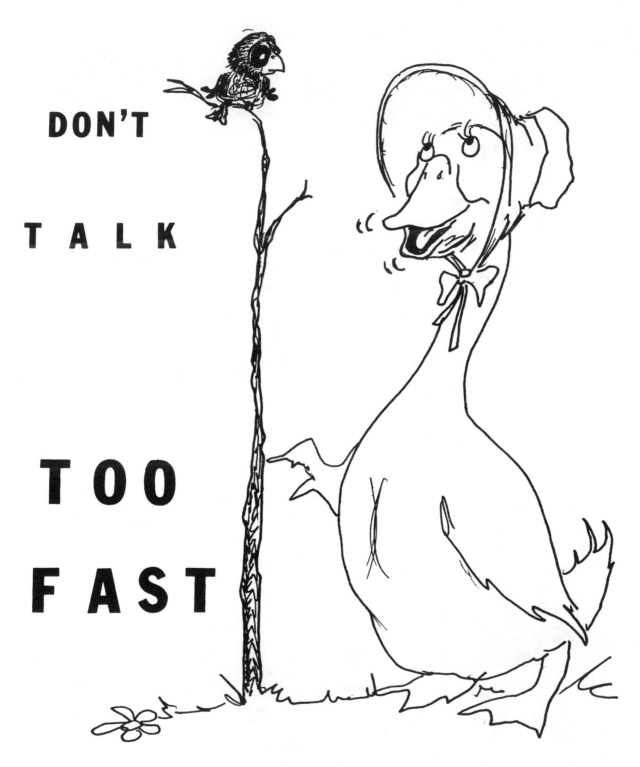

DON'T

TALK

TOO

FAST

Figure 6–13.

Certificate of Achievement

awarded to:

_____

I HAVE COMPLETED THE PROGRAM IN USING MY VOICE CORRECTLY, AND I KNOW HOW TO TAKE CARE OF MY VOICE TO KEEP IT HEALTHY.

_____ Signed

_____ Date

Figure 6–14.

A simple certificate of completion.

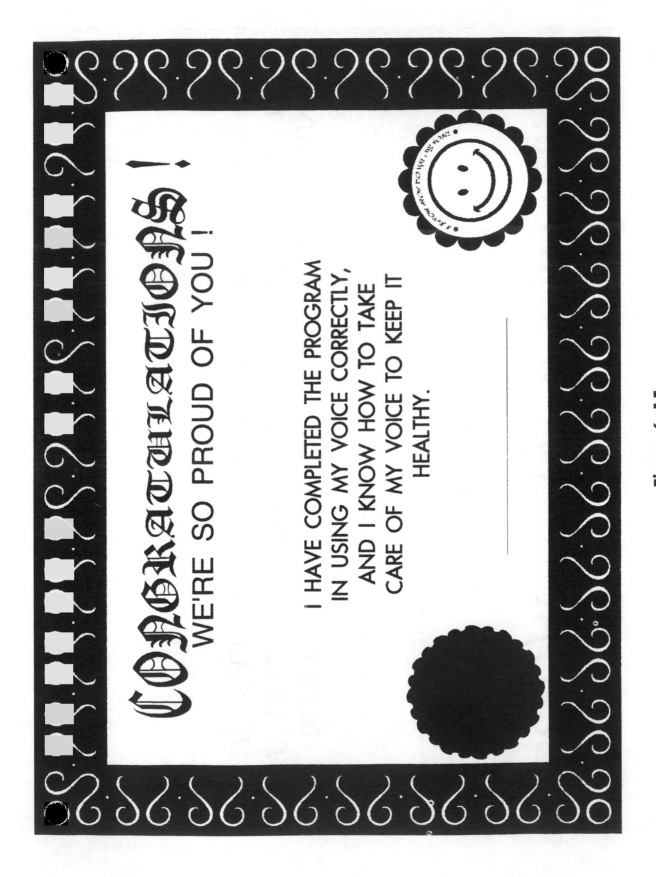

Figure 6–15.

A more ornate certificate of completion.

References

Boone, D. R. (1991). *Is your voice telling on you?* San Diego: Singular Publishing Group.

Boone, D. R. (1993). *The Boone voice program for children.* Austin, TX: Pro-Ed, Inc.

Burk, K. W. (1972). Concepts of clinical management with children presenting voice disturbances. *Journal of the Kansas Speech and Hearing Association*, Spring, 60–66.

Case, J. L. (1996). *Clinical management of voice disorders.* Austin, TX: Pro-Ed, Inc.

Cook, J. V., Palaski, D. J., & Hanson, W. R. (1979). A vocal hygiene program for school-age children. *Language Speech and Hearing Services in Schools, 22,* 156–157.

Dworkin, J. P., & Meleca, R. J. (1997). *Vocal pathologies: Diagnosis, treatment and case studies.* San Diego: Singular Publishing Group.

Harden, J. (1986). Voice disorders in children [Abstract]. *Asha, 28,* 164.

Kahane, J. C., & Mayo, R. (1989). The need for aggressive pursuit of healthy childhood voices. *Language Speech and Hearing Services in Schools, 20,* 102–107.

Moran, M. J., & Pentz, A. L. (1987). Otolaryngologists' opinions of voice therapy for vocal nodules in children. *Language Speech and Hearing Services in Schools, 18,* 172–178.

Mutch, P. (1976). *Hoarseness among school children in proximity to a source of air pollution.* Master's thesis, University of Florida.

Nilson, H., & Schneiderman, C. R. (1983). Classroom program for the prevention of vocal abuse and hoarseness in elementary school children. *Language Speech and Hearing Services in Schools, 14,* 121–127.

Sander, E. K. (1989). Arguments against the aggressive pursuit of voice therapy for children. *Language Speech and Hearing Services in Schools, 20,* 94–101.

Sauchelli, K. (1979). *The incidence of hoarseness among school-age children in a pollution-free community.* Master's thesis, University of Florida.

Senturia, B., & Wilson, F. (1968). Otorhinolaryngic findings in children with voice deviations. *Annals of Otology, Rhinology, and Laryngology, 77,* 1027–1041.

Stasney, C. R. (1996). *Atlas of dynamic laryngeal pathology.* San Diego: Singular Publishing Group.

Stemple, J. C., Glaze, L. E., & Gerdeman, B. K. (1995). *Clinical voice pathology: Theory and management* (2nd ed.). San Diego: Singular Publishing Group.

Terrell, S. L., & Morgan, P. A. (1980). *The adventures of Mr. Gruff: A voice therapy program for pre-school children.* Paper presented to the annual convention of the American Speech-Language-Hearing Association, Detroit, MI.

Wilson, D. K. (1987). *Voice problems of children* (3rd ed.). Baltimore: Williams & Wilkins.

Wilson, F. B. (1972). The voice disordered child: A descriptive approach. *Language Speech and Hearing Services in Schools, 4,* 14–22.

List of Photographs

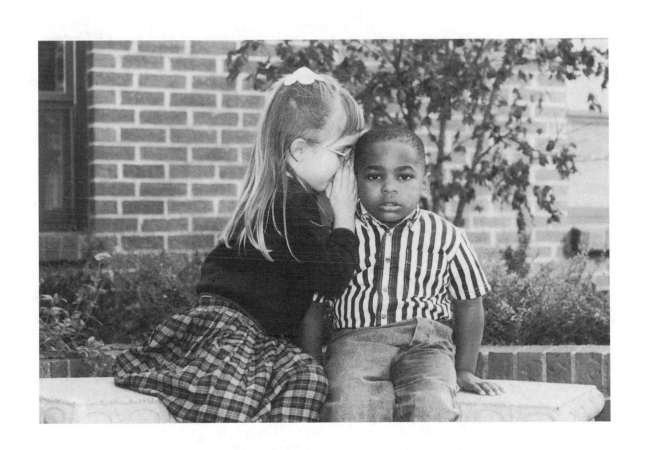

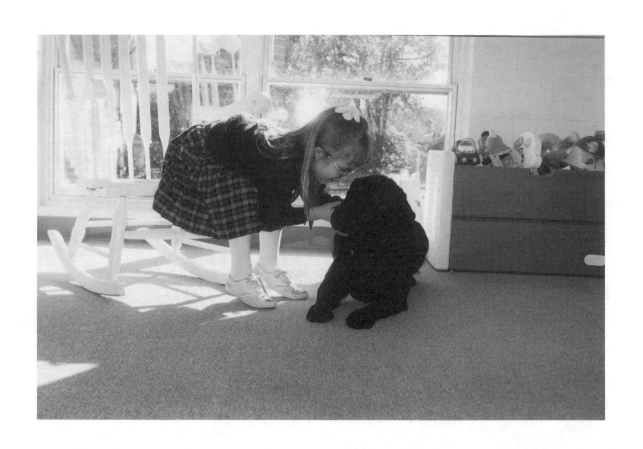

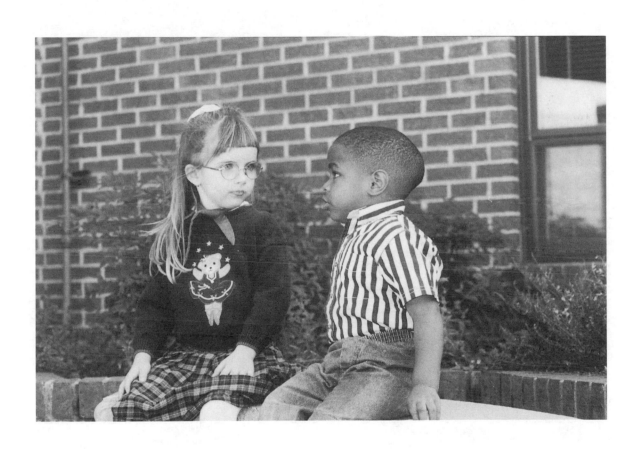

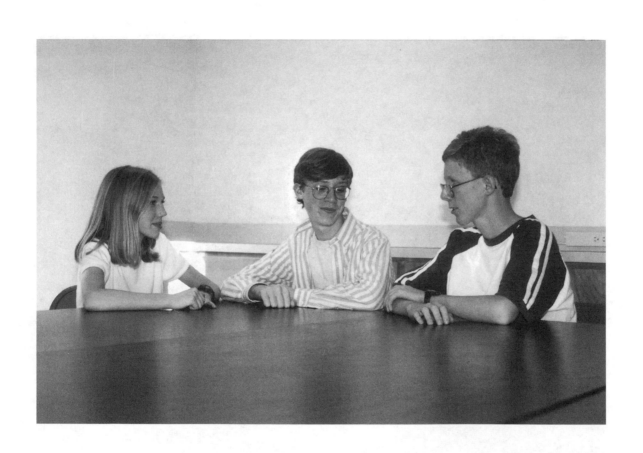

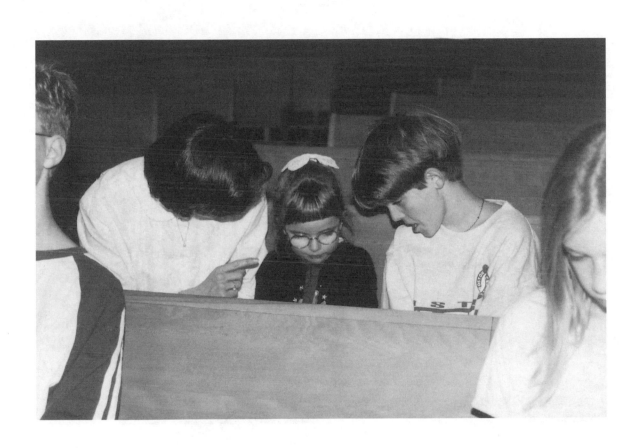

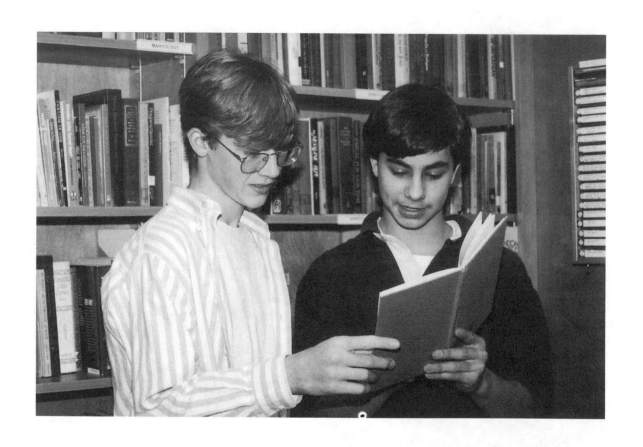

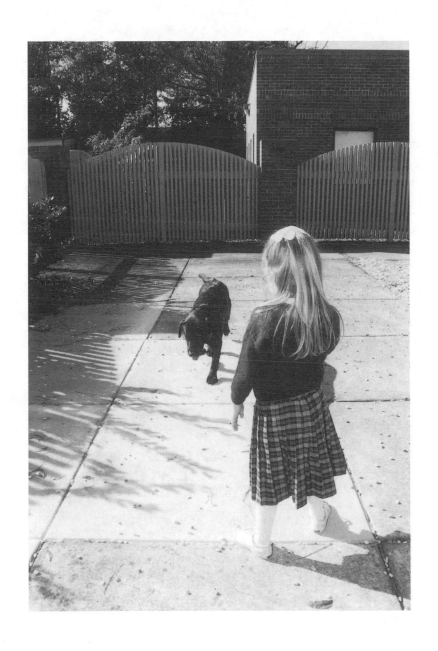

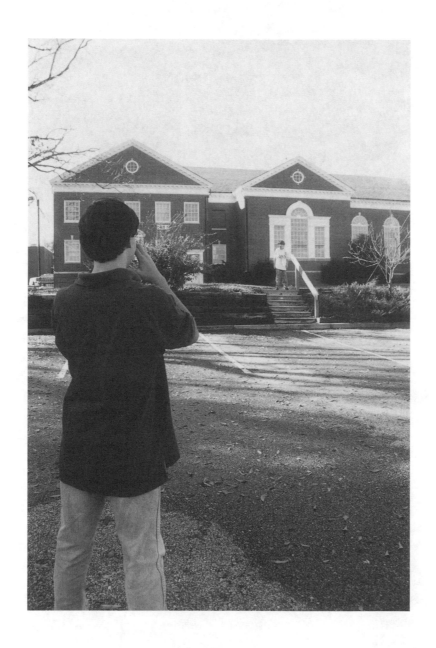

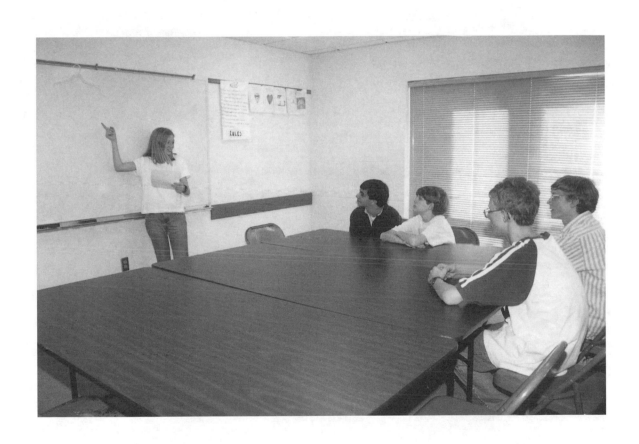

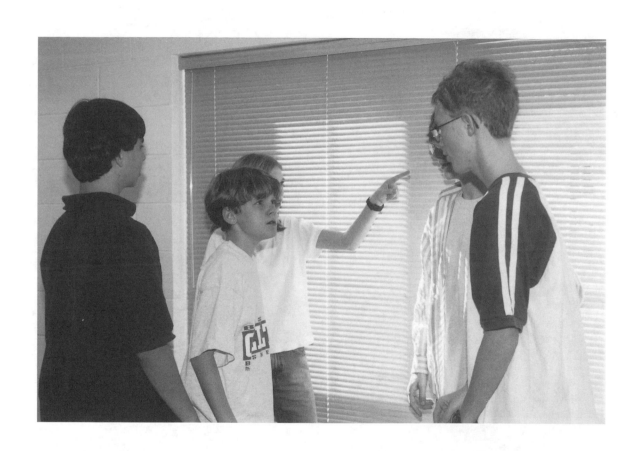

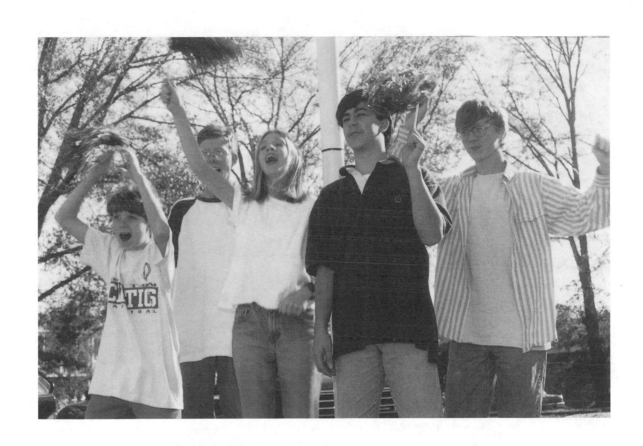

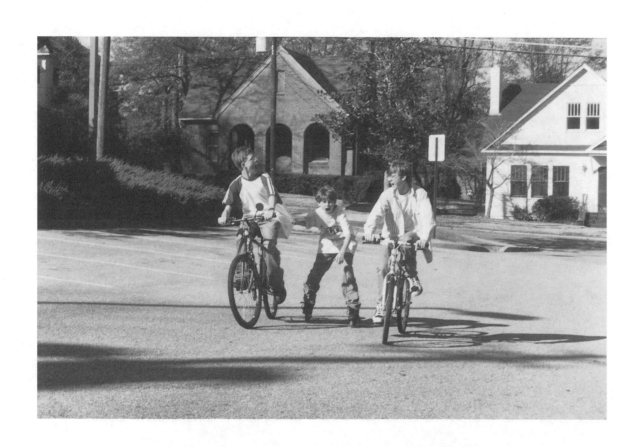

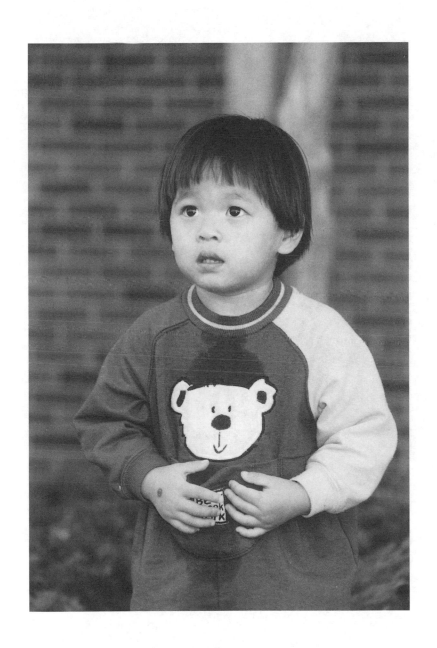

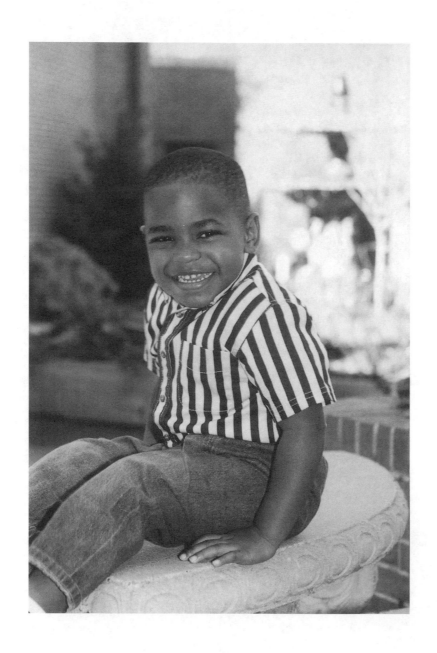

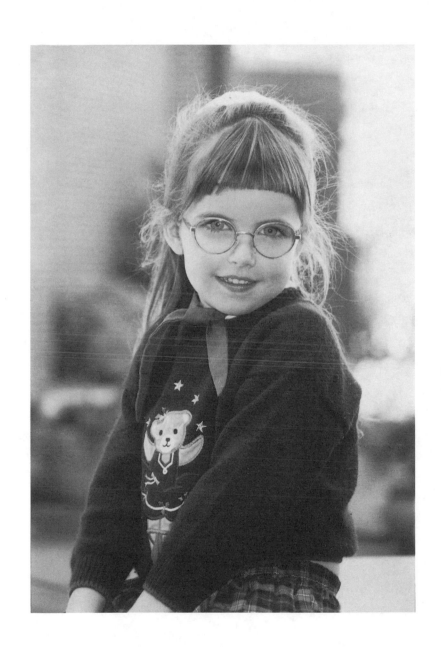

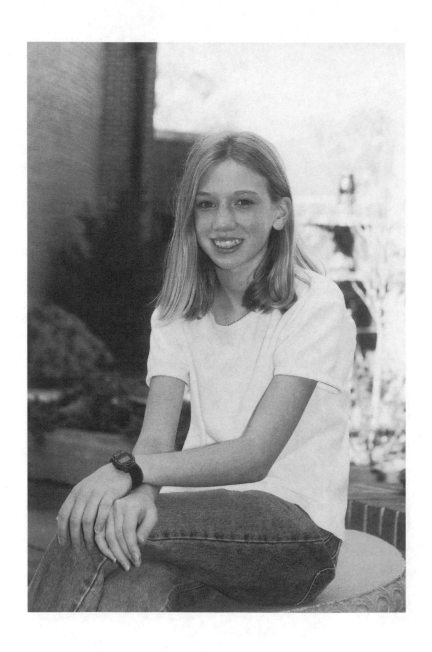

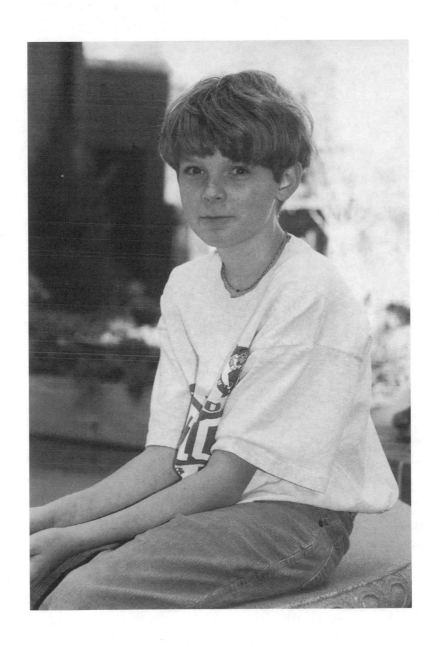

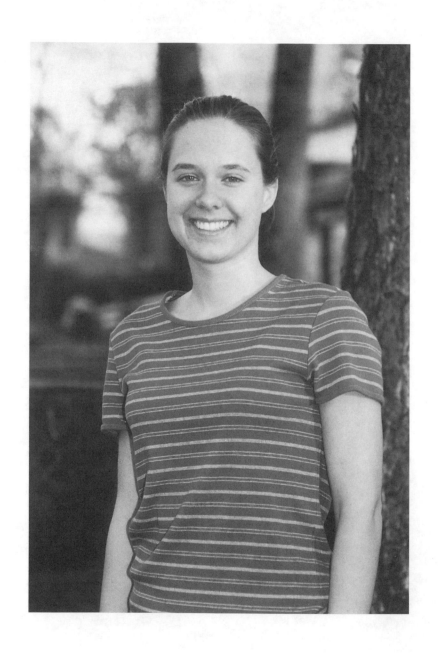

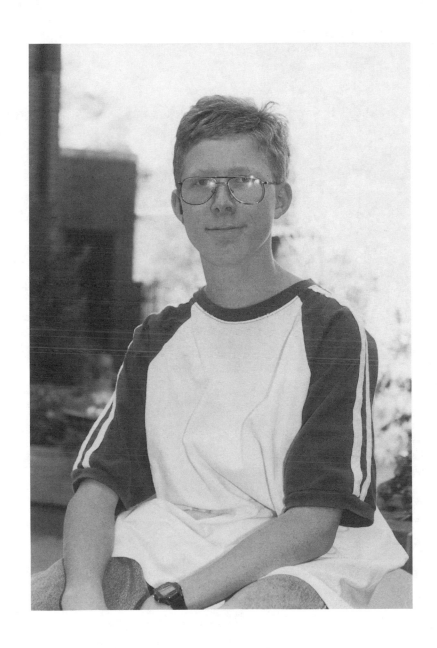

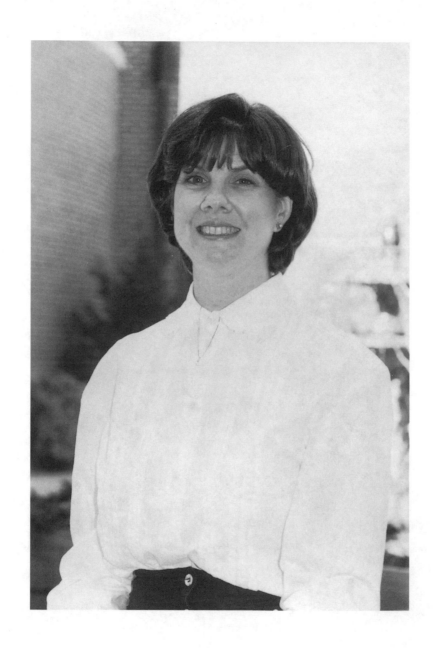

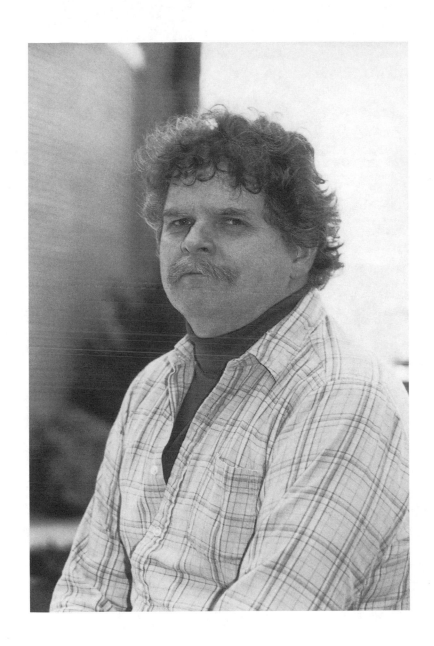

Index